How do you like ou

We would really appreciate you leaving us a review.

MW01224939

Other Picture Books:

For other fun Picture Books by Kampelstone,
simply search for:

Kampelstone Picture Books

Scotland facts

- The national animal of Scotland is the unicorn.

- Scotland has the highest number of redheads per capita than anywhere else in the world. One out of every 8 people there have red hair.

- Scots have a higher percentage of blue eyes than those in the rest of Britain. In the Southeast of Scotland, the percentage is nearly 60%.

- The tallest hedge in the world is in Meikleour, Scotland. It is 100 feet (30 meters) high and more than 1700 feet (518 meters) long.

- The oldest tree in Europe is in Scotland. The Fortingall Yew is about 3000 years old.

- Golf was invented in Scotland and St. Andrews Links is the 'home of golf'. Golf has been played in Scotland since the 1400's.

- Scotland also has the shortest commercial flight in the world. When traveling from Westray to Papa Westray in Orkney, the flight lasts about ¾ of a minute.

- Of Scotland's 790 islands, only 130 are inhabited.

- The longest ever reverberation of an echo was made inside Inchindown tunnels. It was a fuel-storage facility near Invergordon in Ross-shire built during WWII. From the report of a fired gun, the reverberating echo lasted the better part of two minutes.

- There are as many people with Scottish heritage living in the United States as there are Scots in Scotland.

- Scotland has three officially recognized languages: English, Scots and Scottish Gaelic.

- Edinburgh is the first city in the world to have a municipal fire brigade. Its brigade was organized in 1703.

- Bonnybridge, a small town in Scotland, has become, like Roswell, a UFO capital of the world. There are more than 300 sightings of UFOs reported every year.

- Alexander Graham Bell, a Scotsman, invented the telephone in February 1876 and a fellow Scot, John Logie Baird, created the first TV picture in October 1925.

- The tallest waterfall in Britain, named Eas a' Chual Aluinn, has a drop of 658 feet (200 meters) twice as high as Victoria Falls.

- Scotland has over 600 square miles (1550 square kilometers) of freshwater lakes.

- The Macintosh raincoat was invented in Scotland by Charles Macintosh from Glasgow.

- Scotland is famous for its single-malt whisky. The word "whisky" comes from Old Irish 'uisce beatha' which means "water of life."

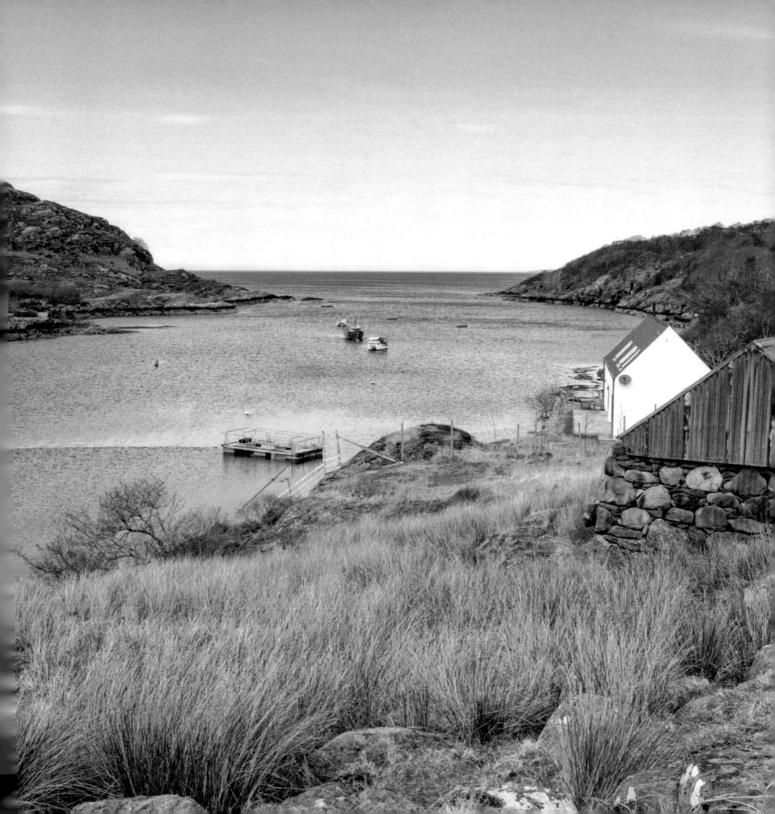

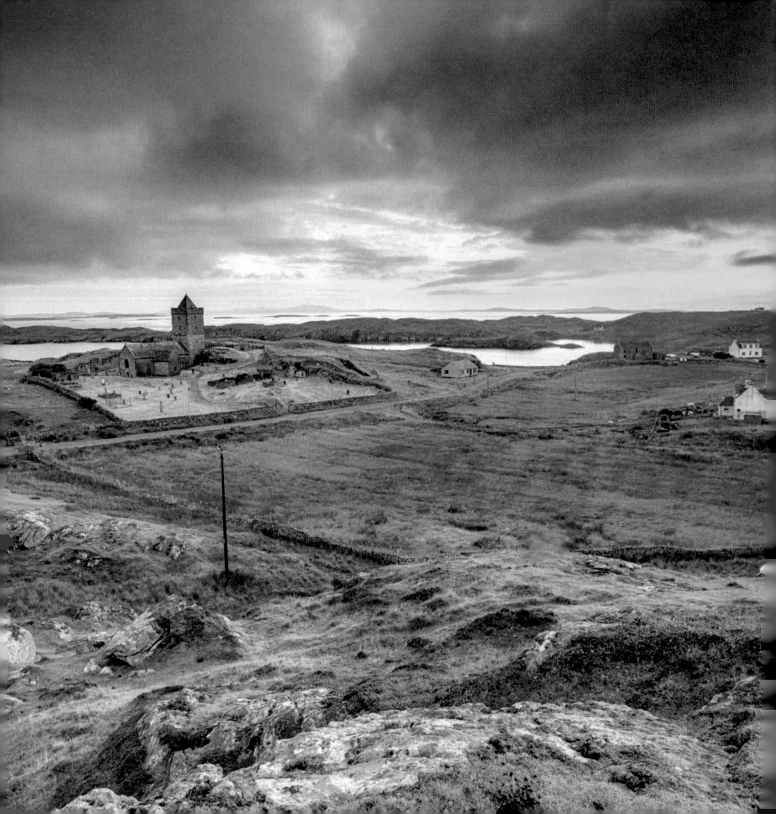

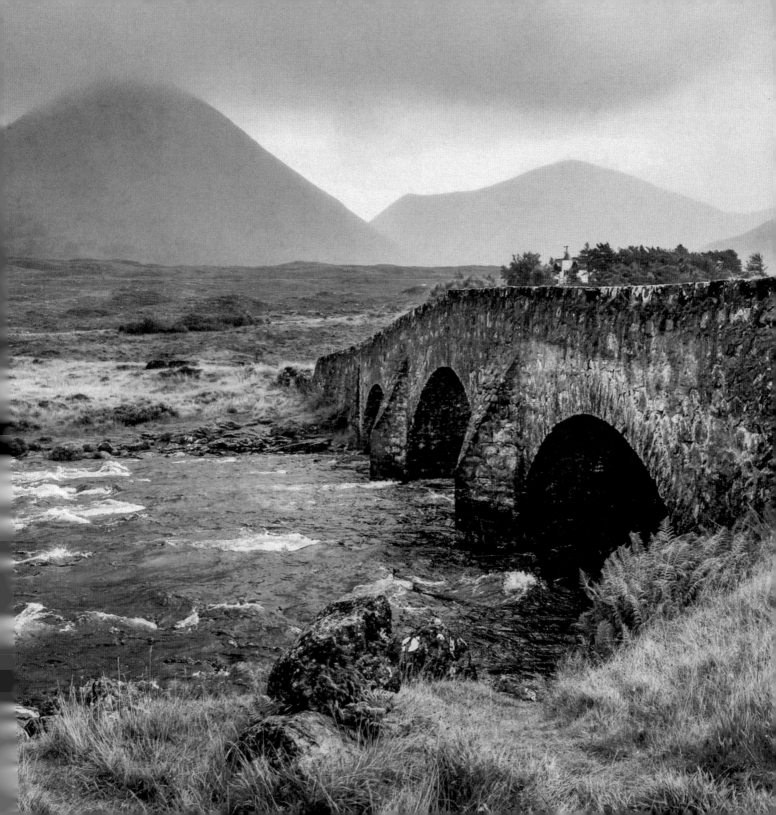

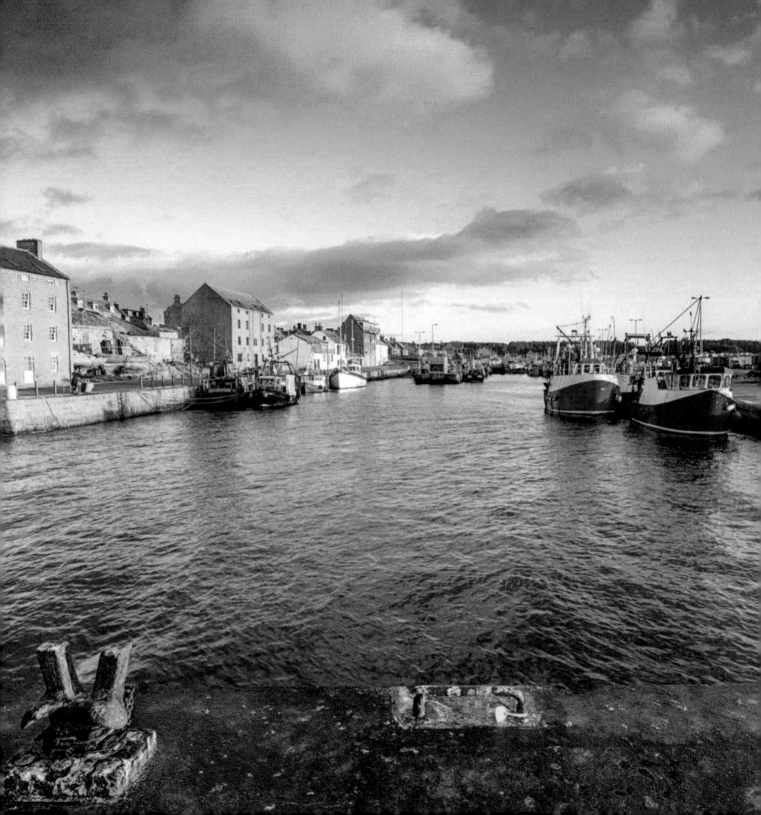

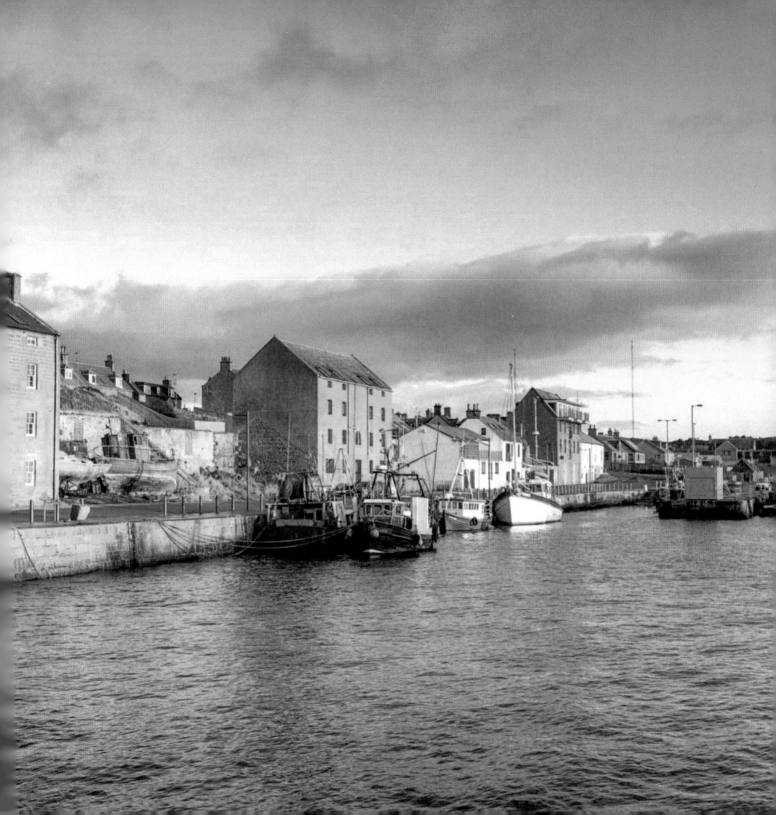

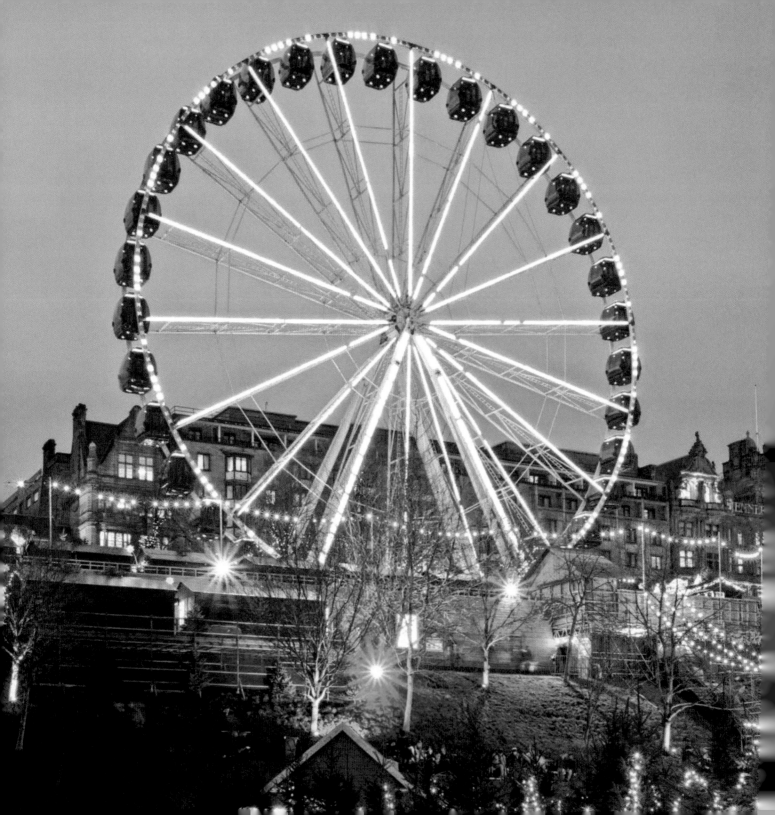

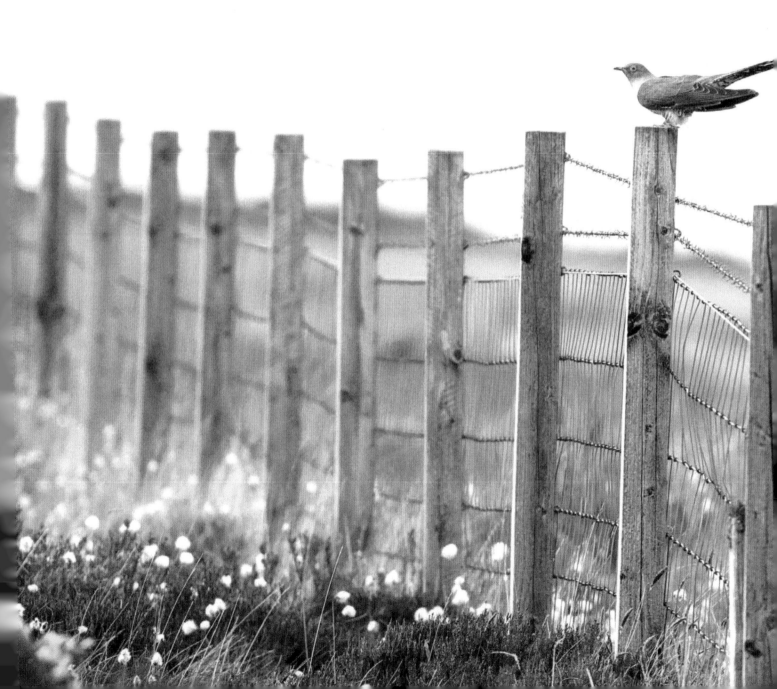

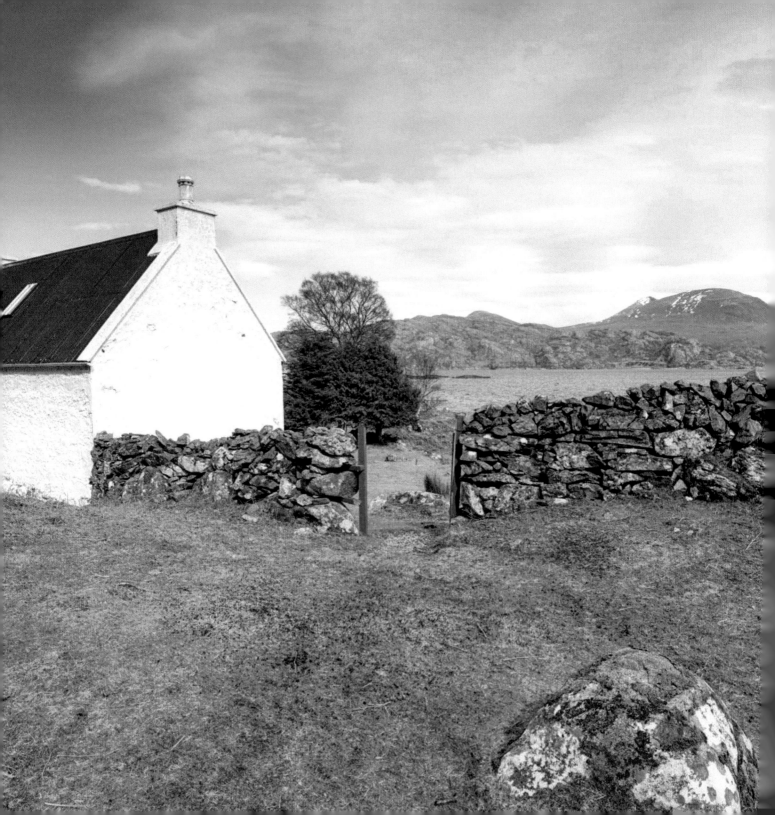

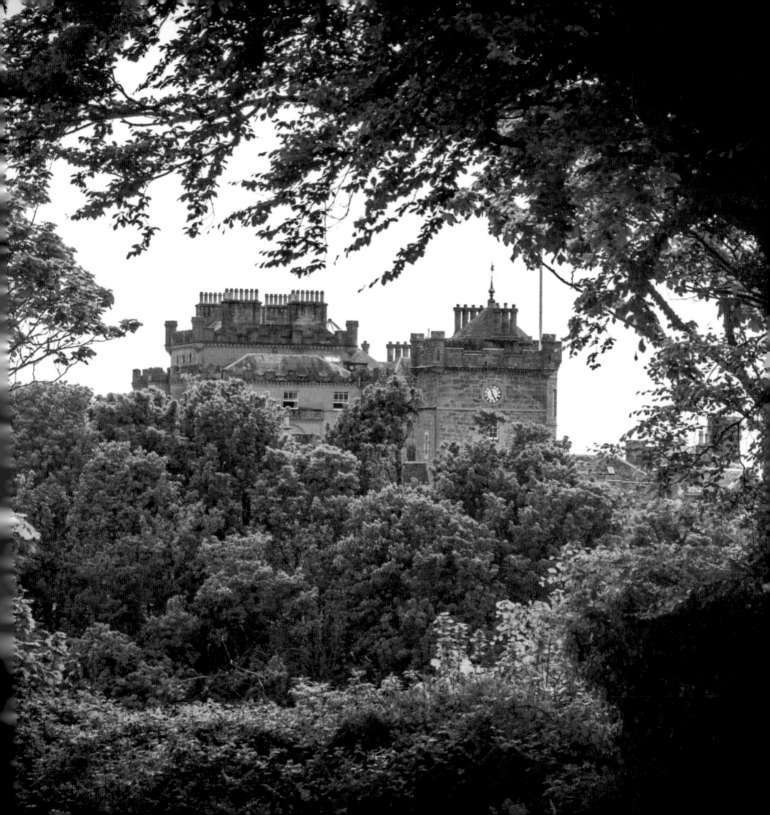

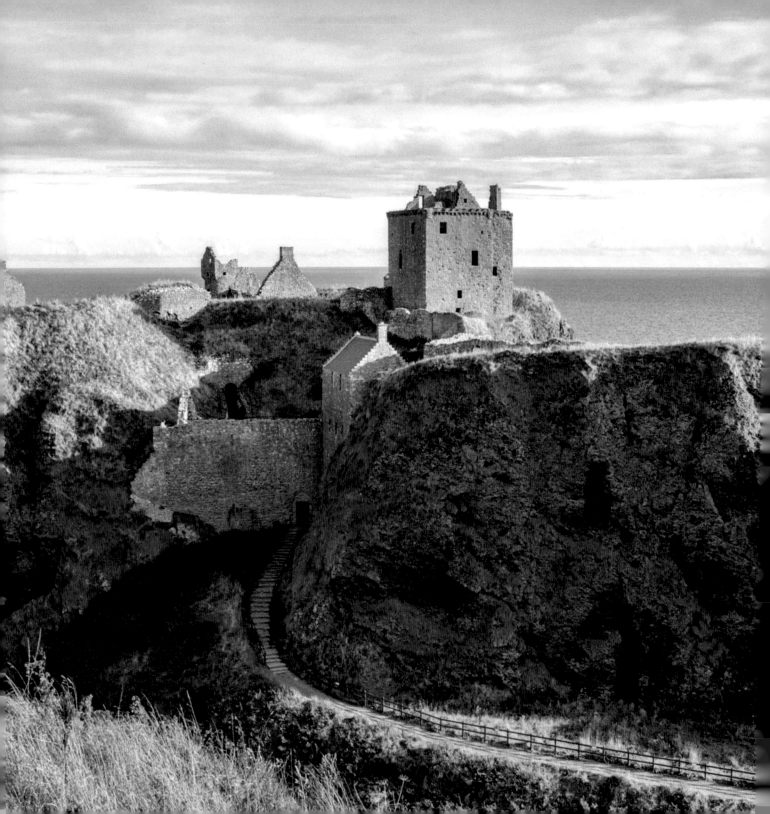

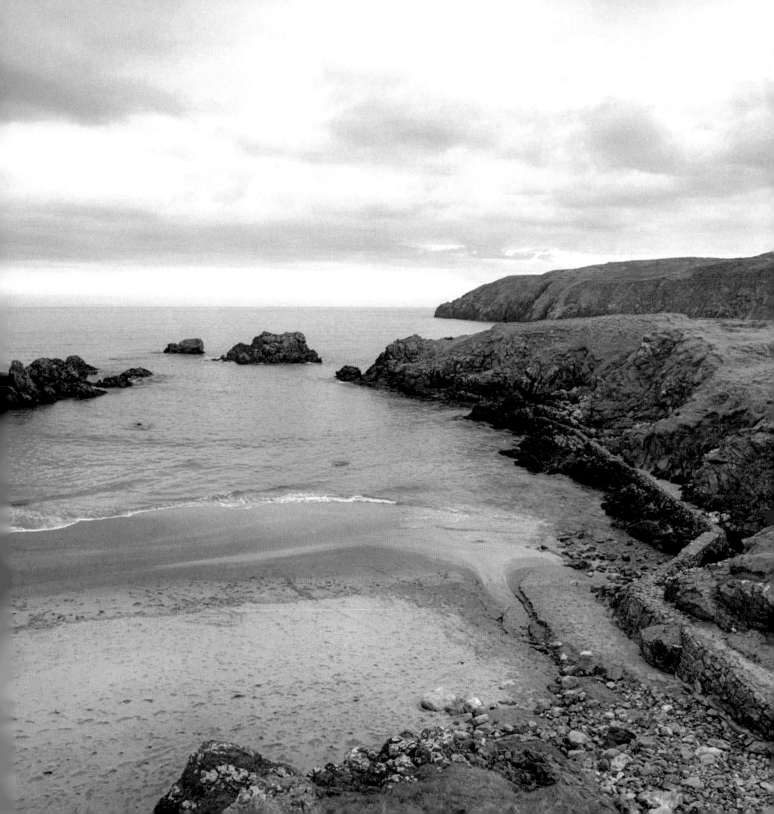

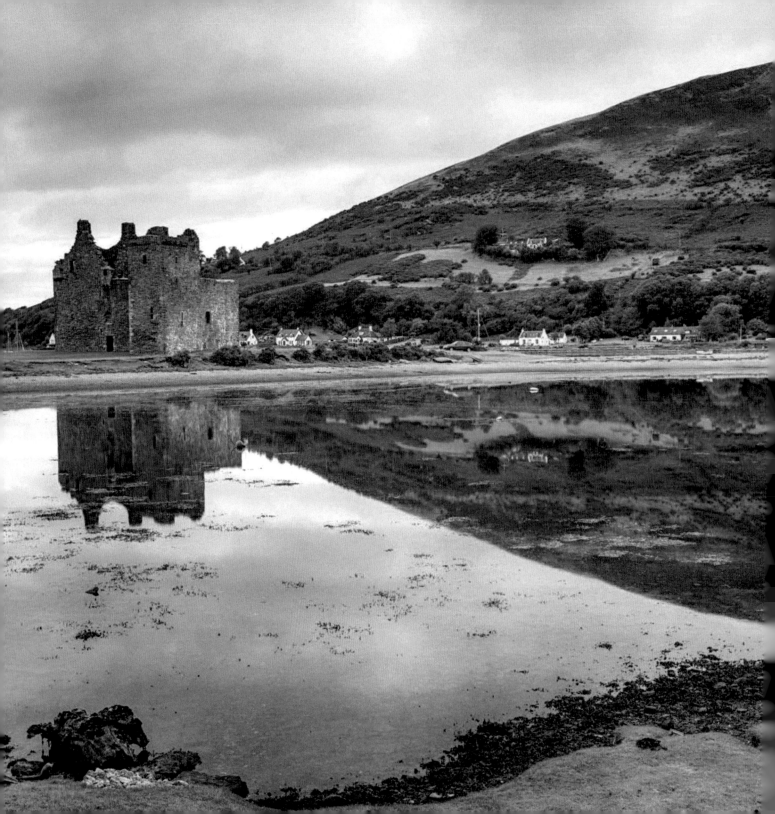

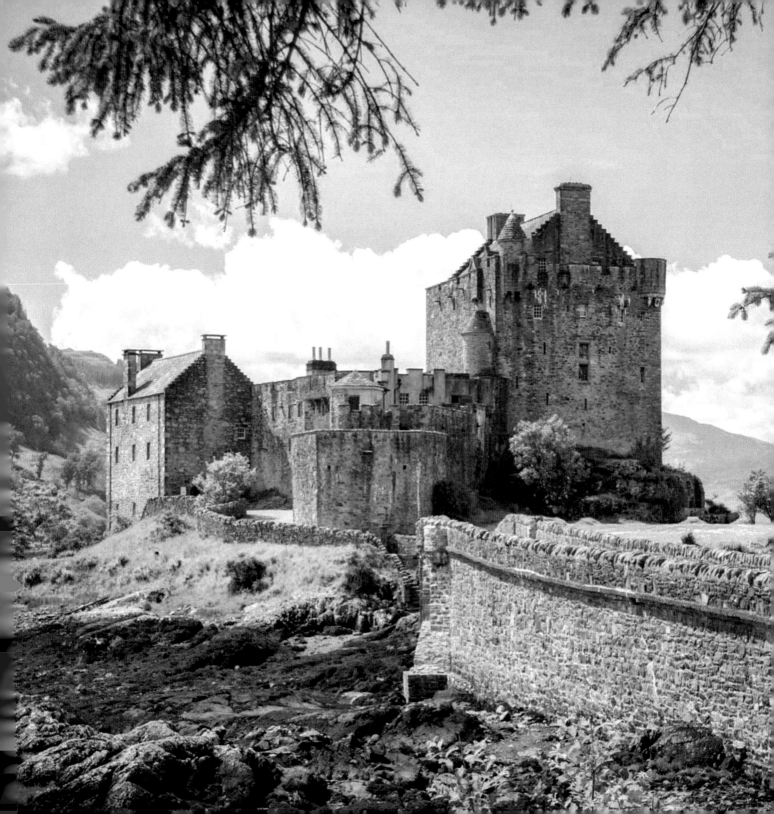

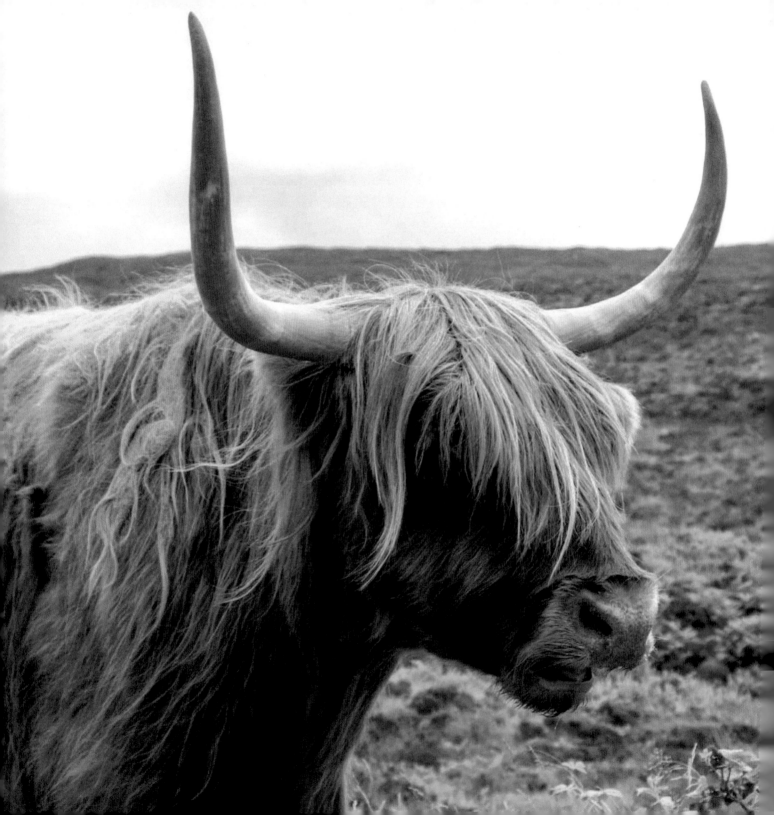

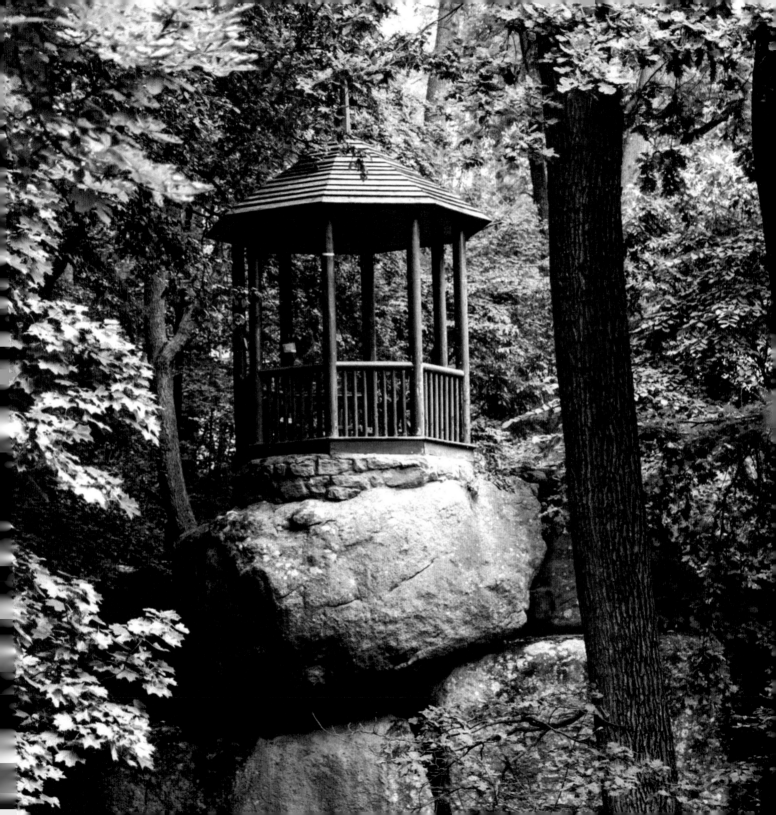

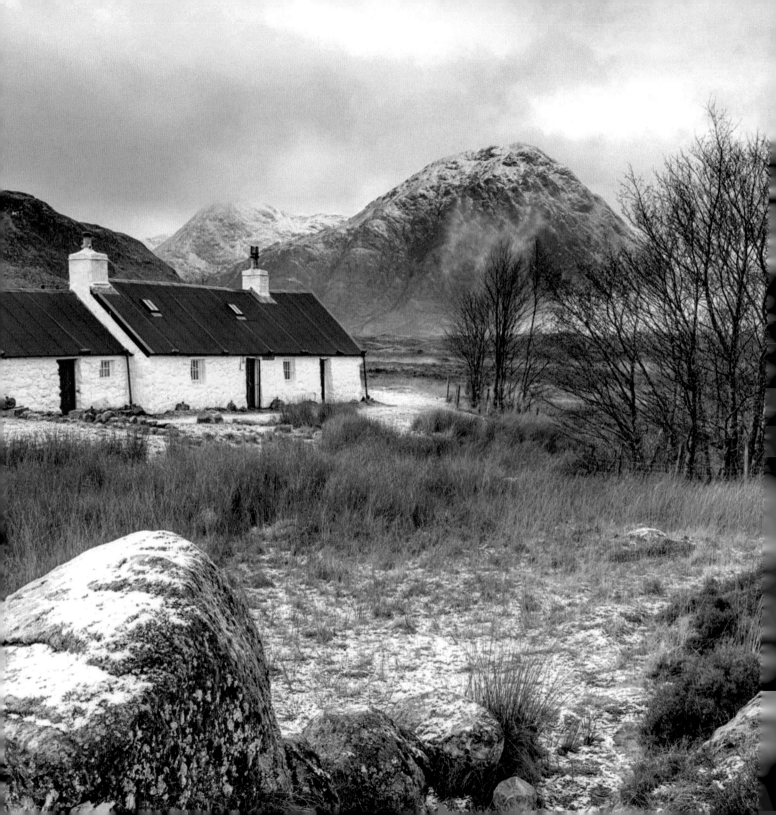

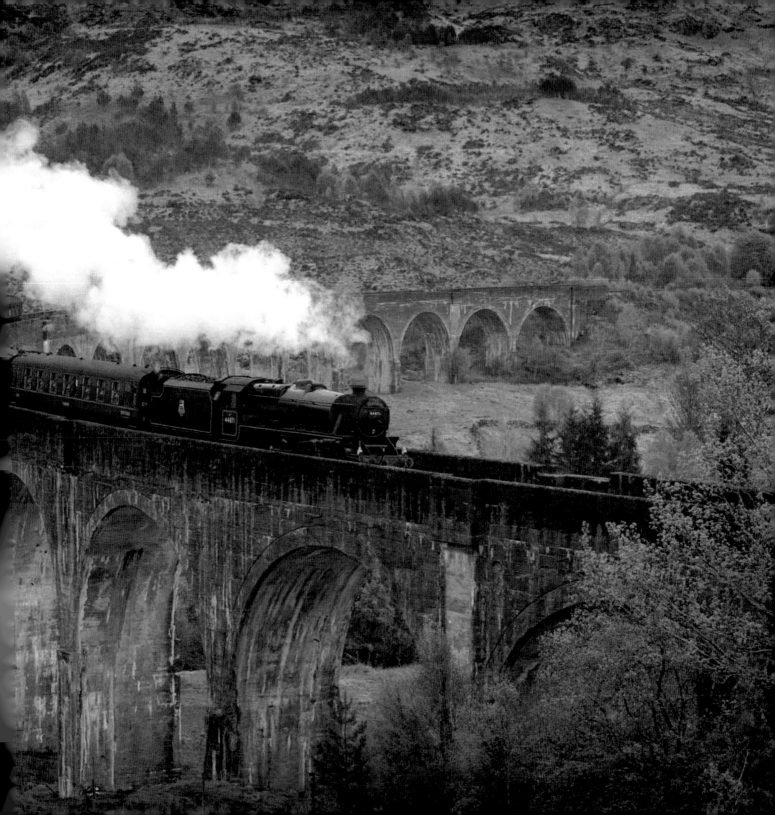

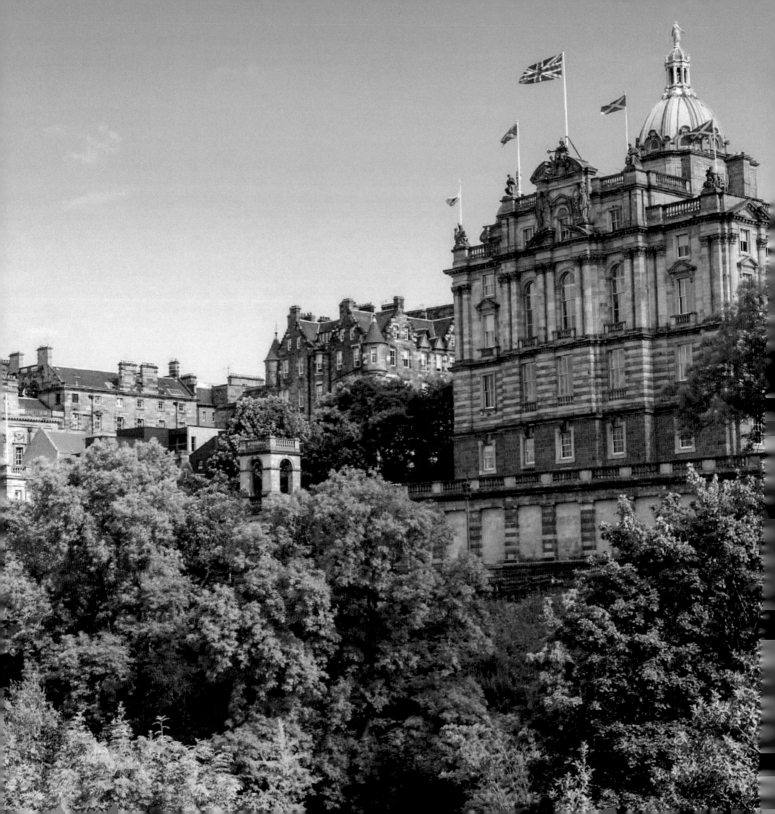

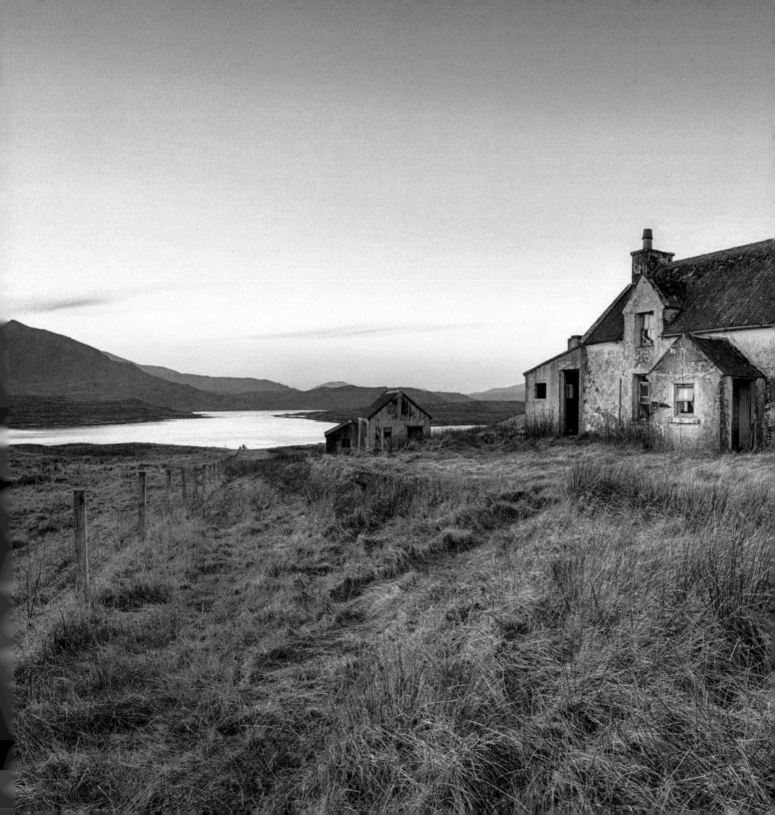

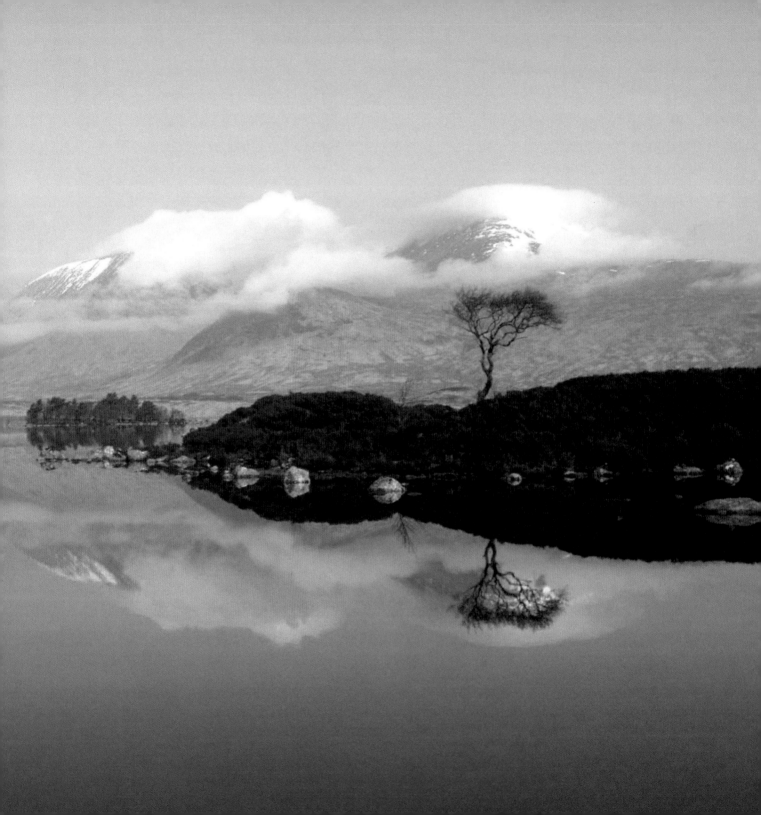

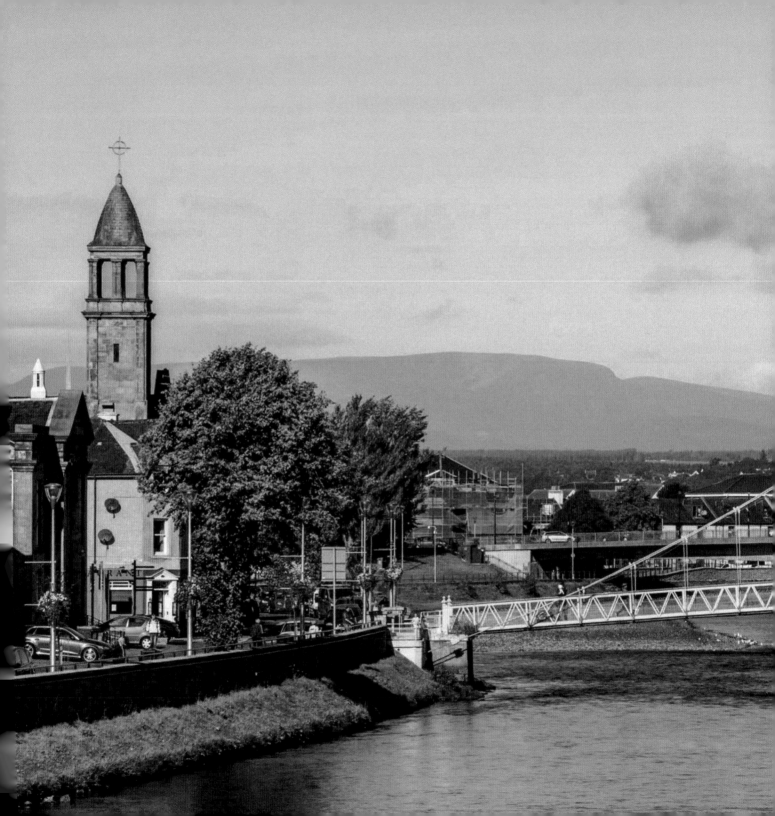

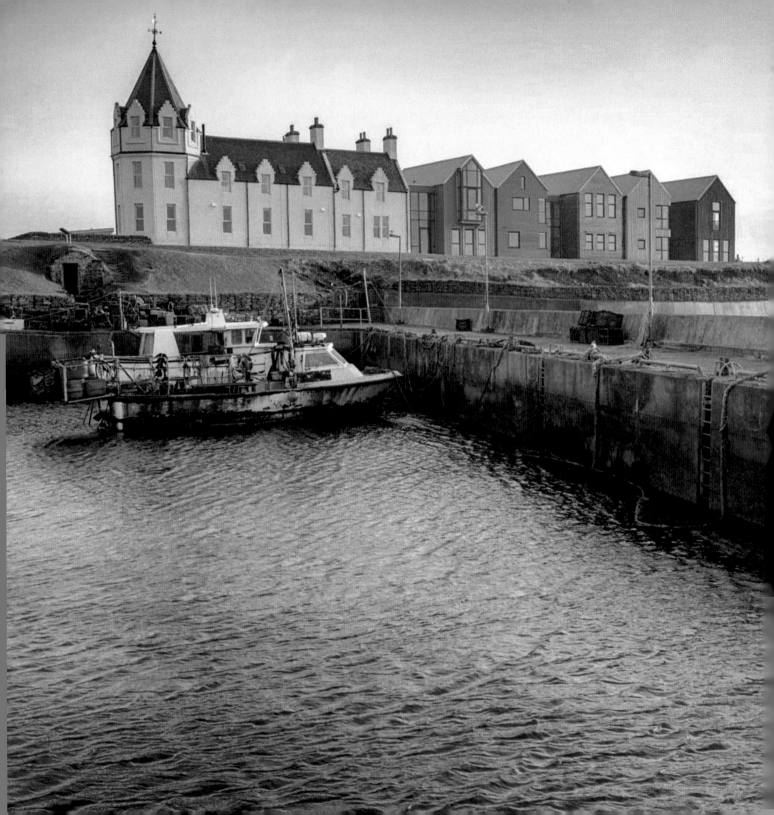

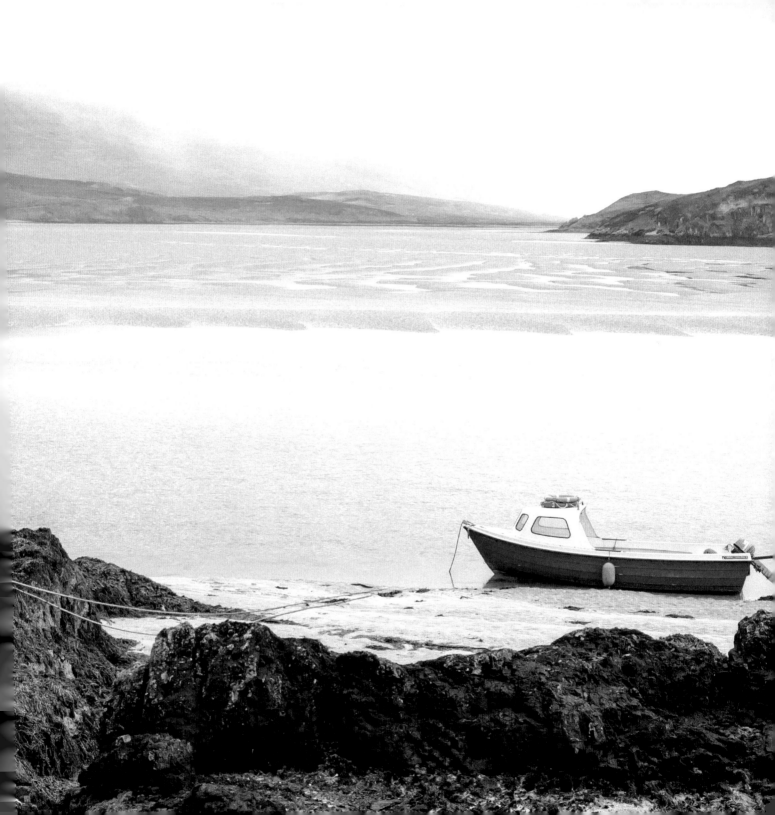

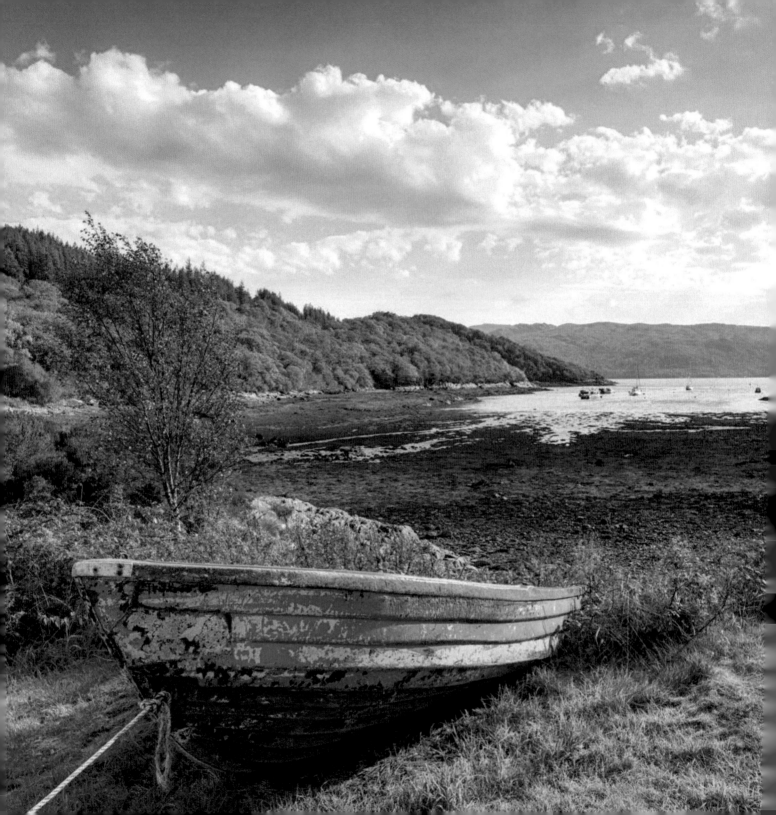

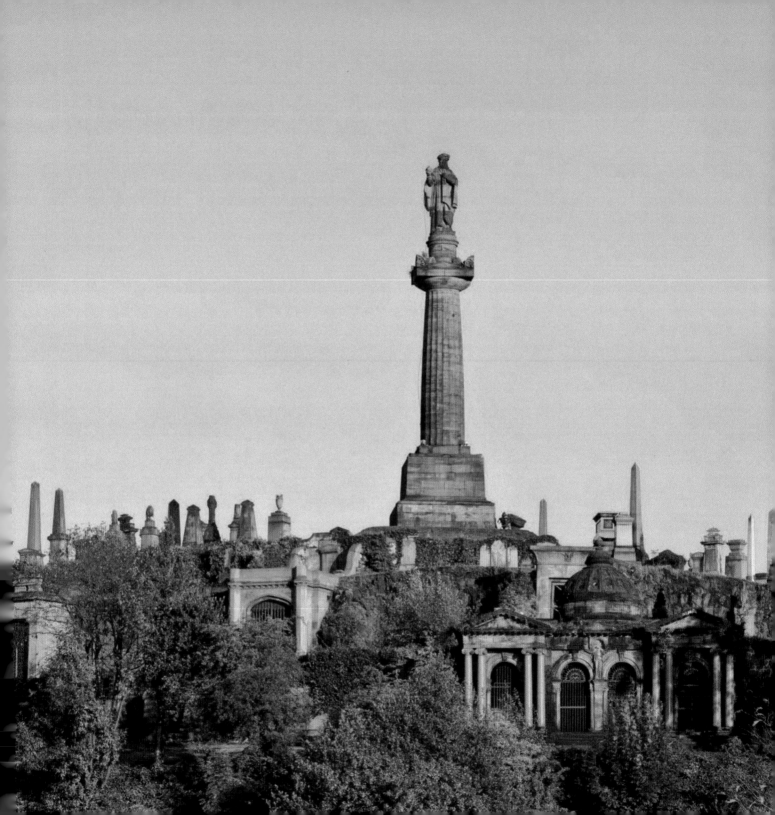

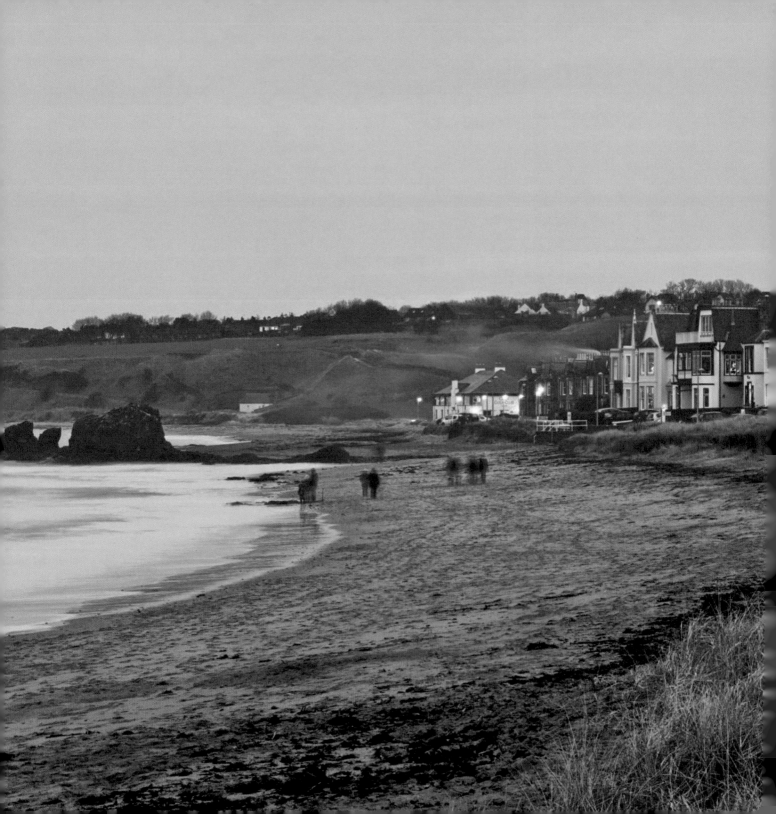

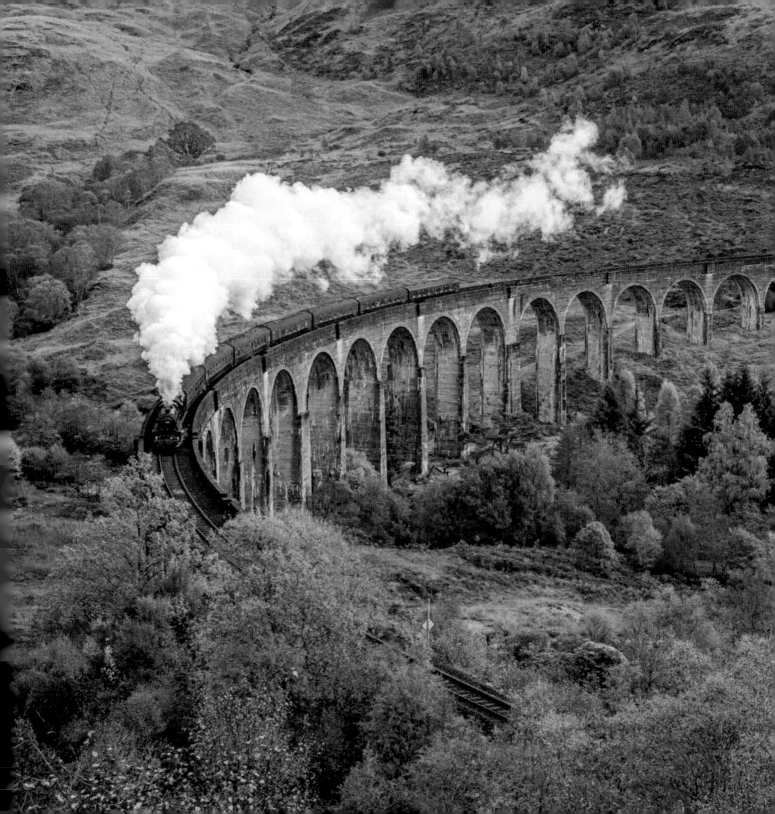

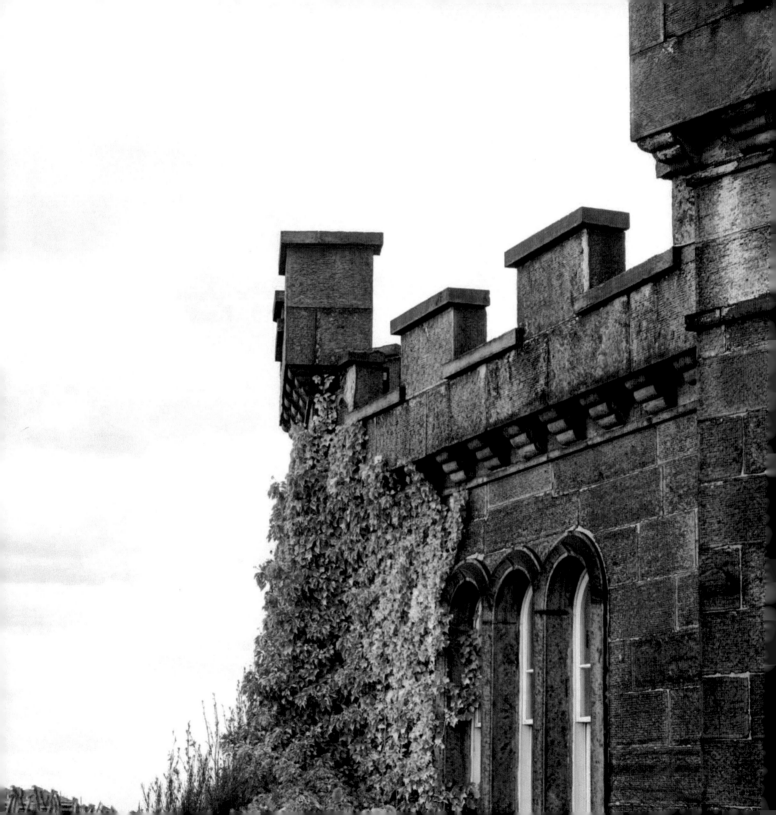

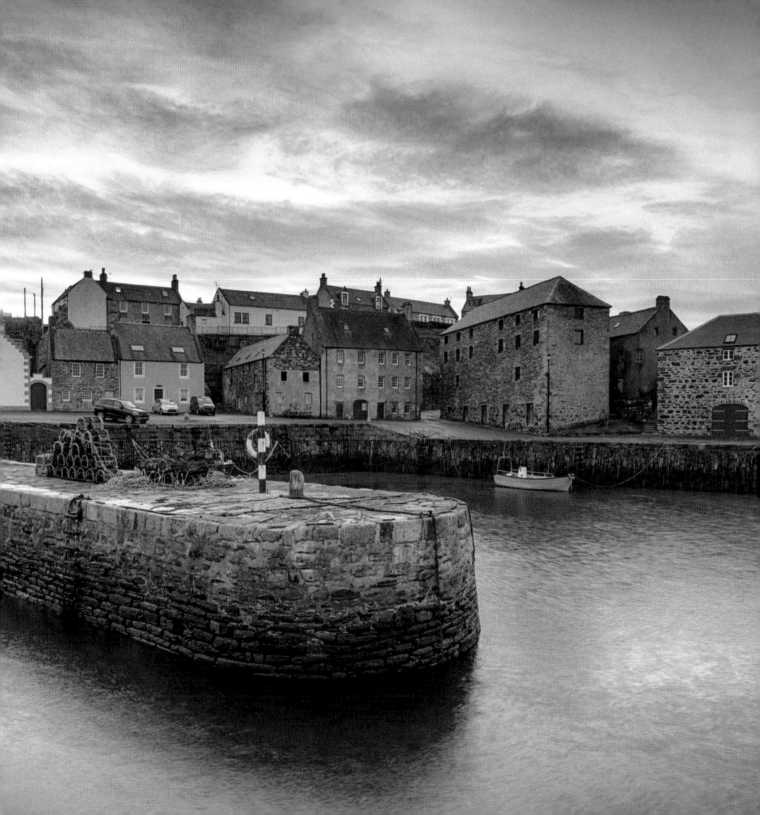

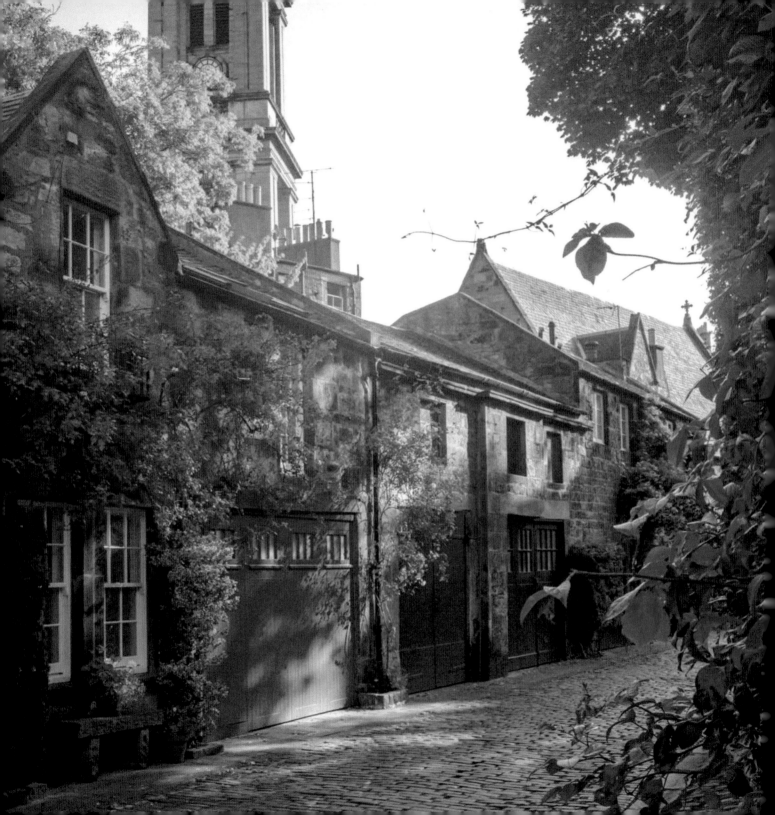

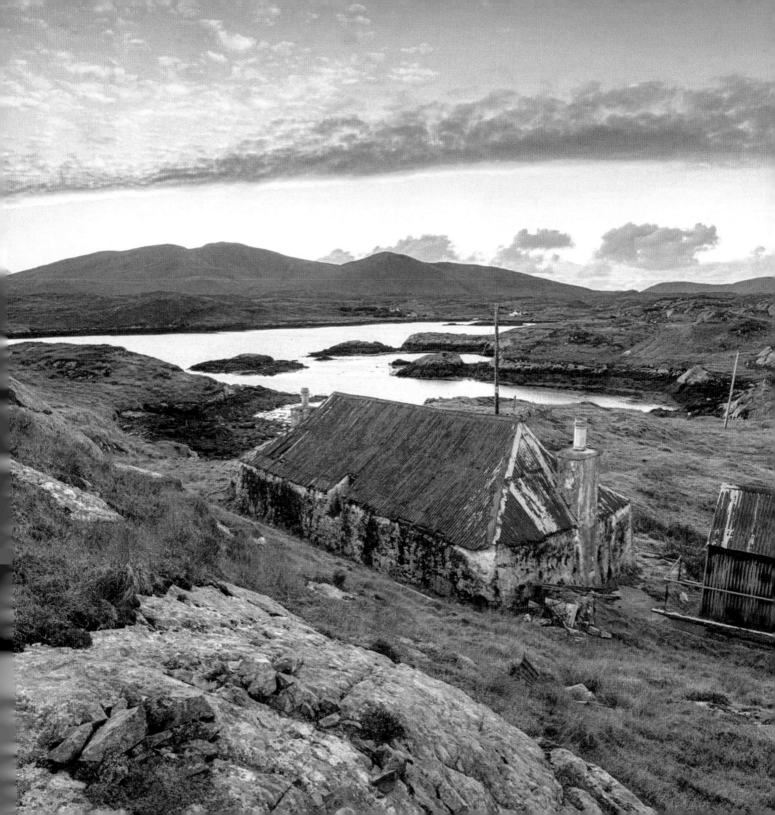

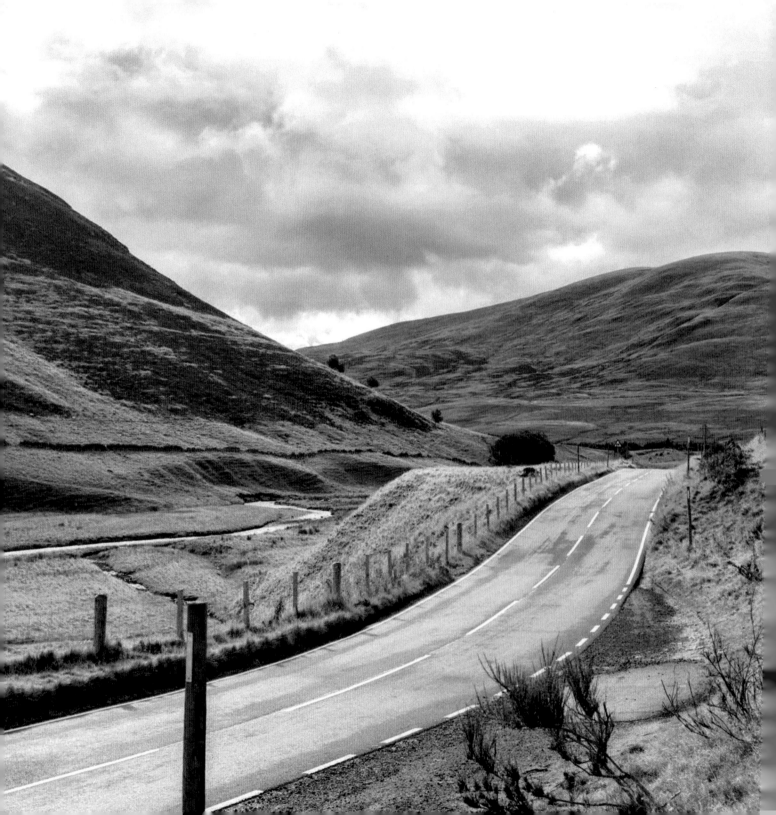

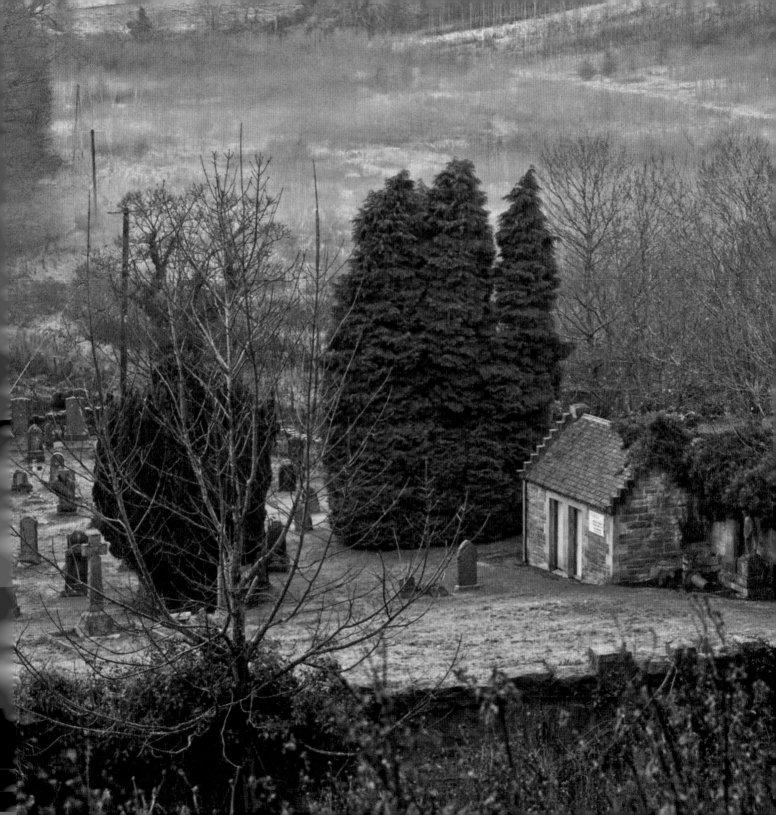

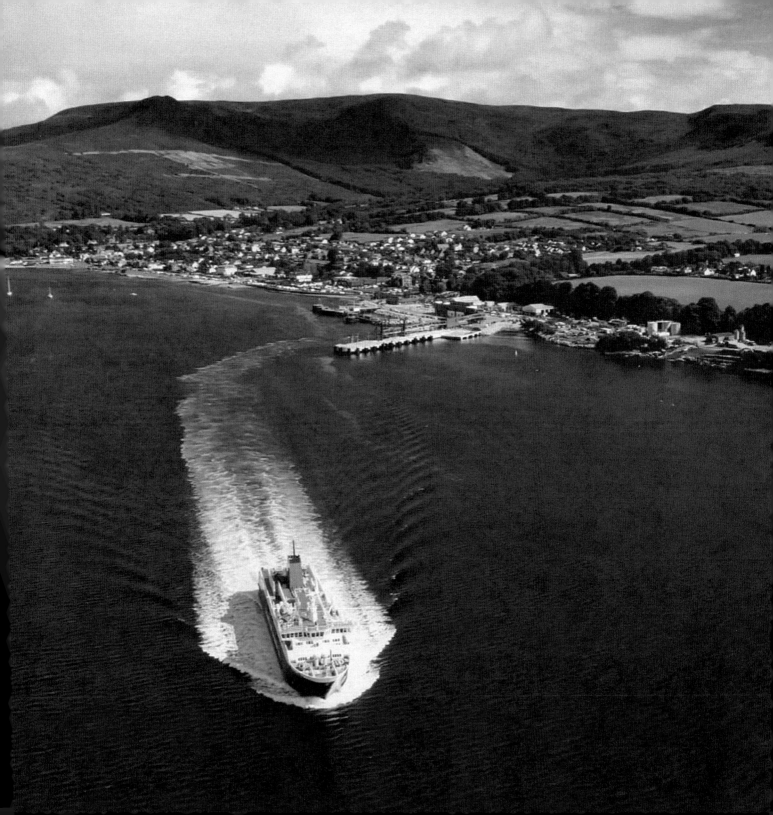

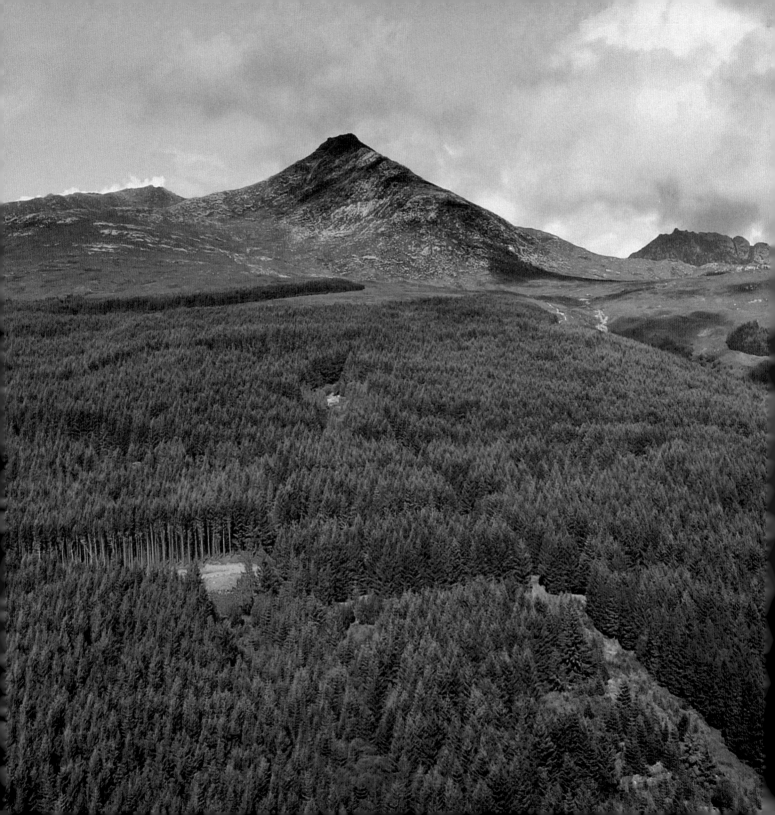

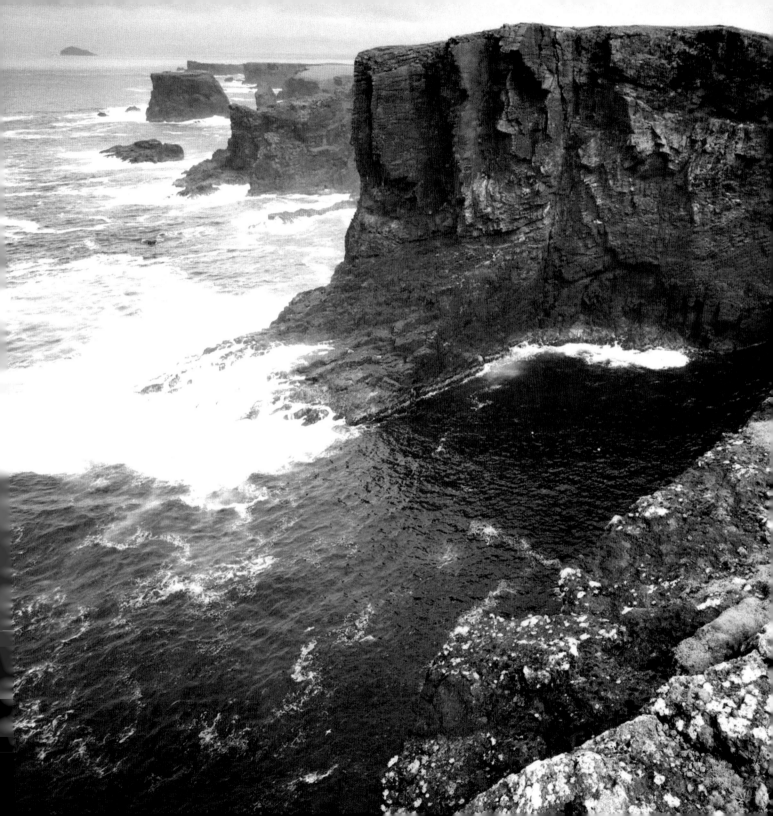

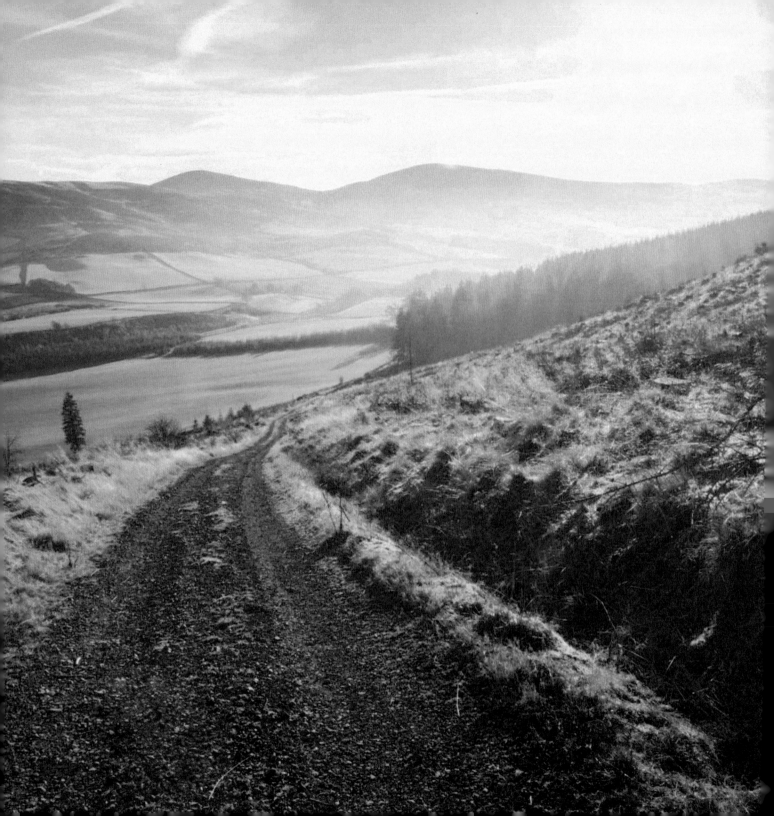

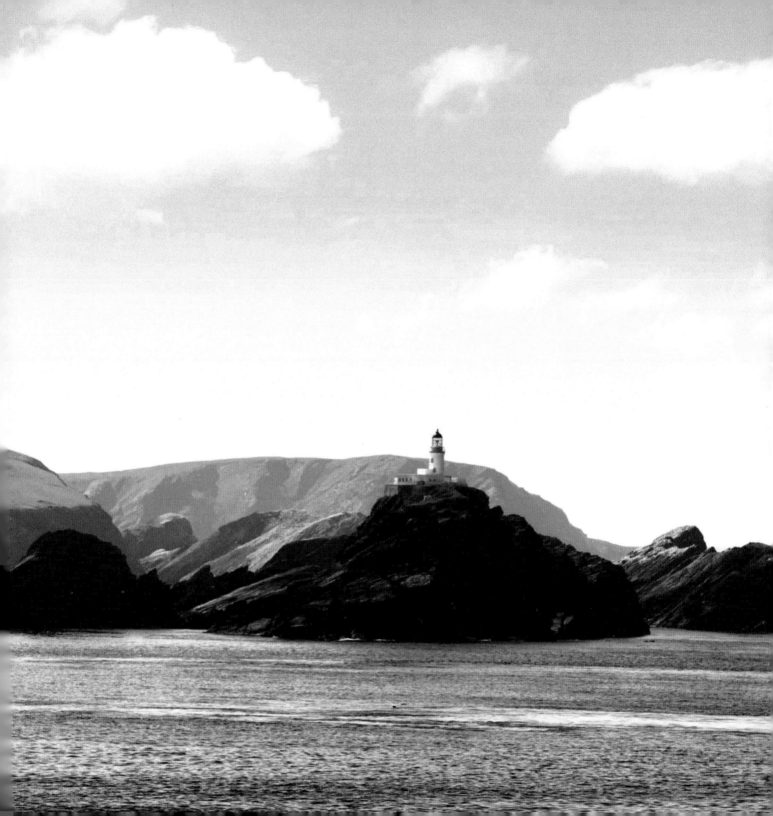

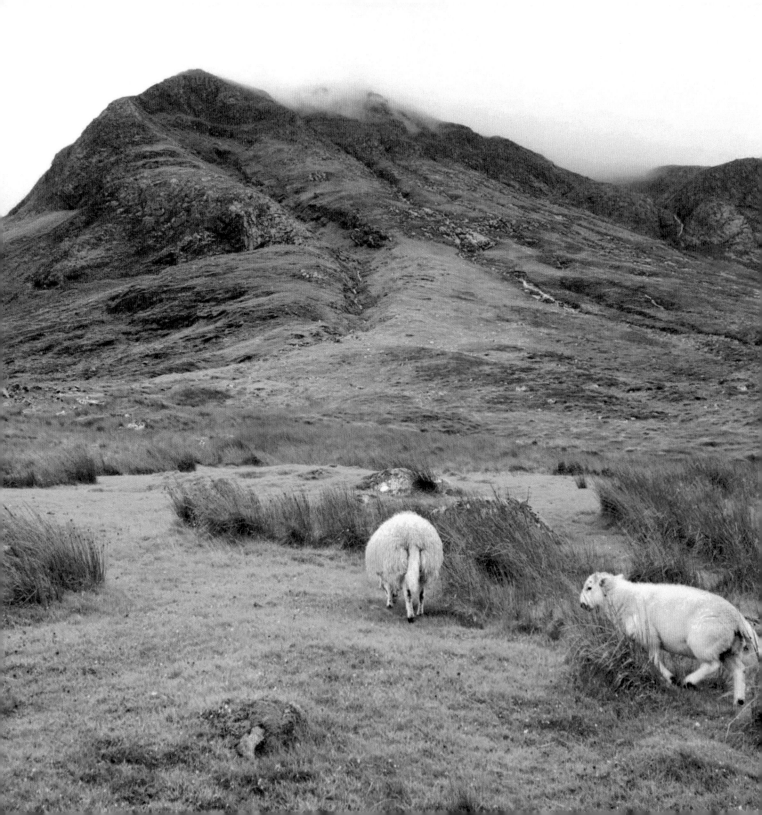

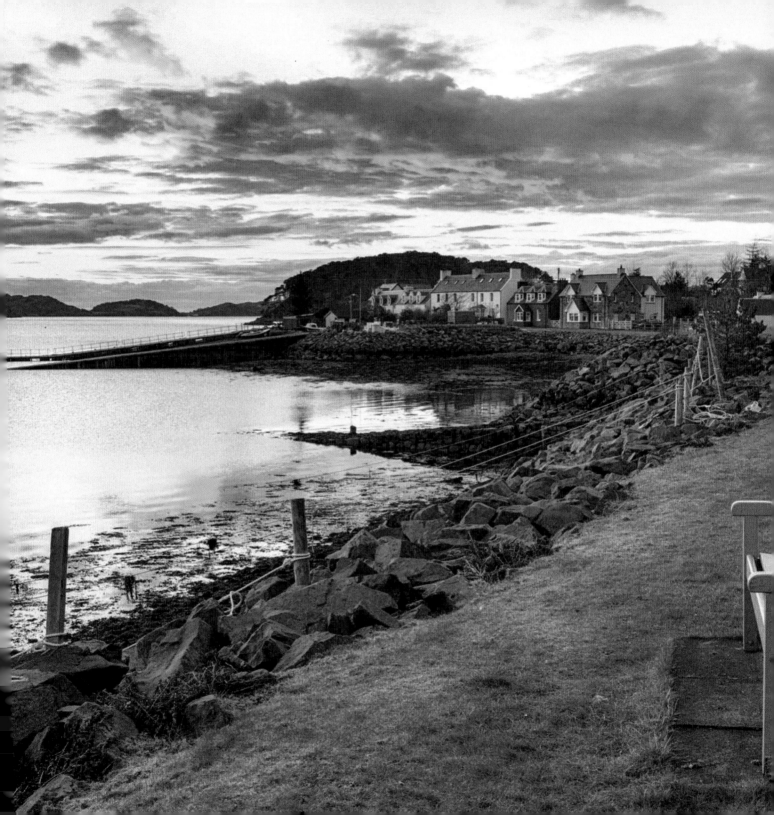

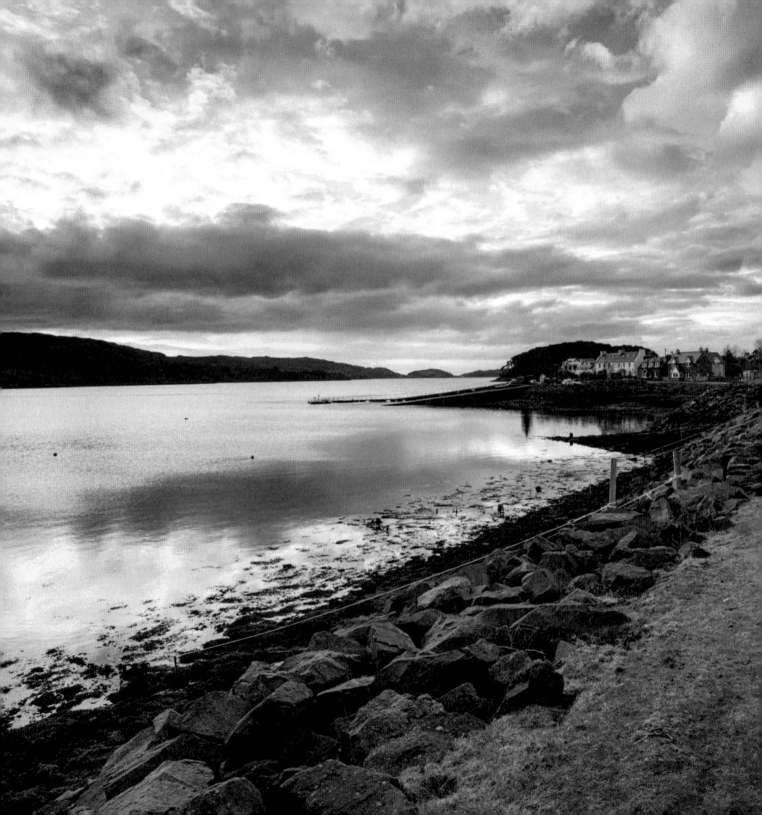

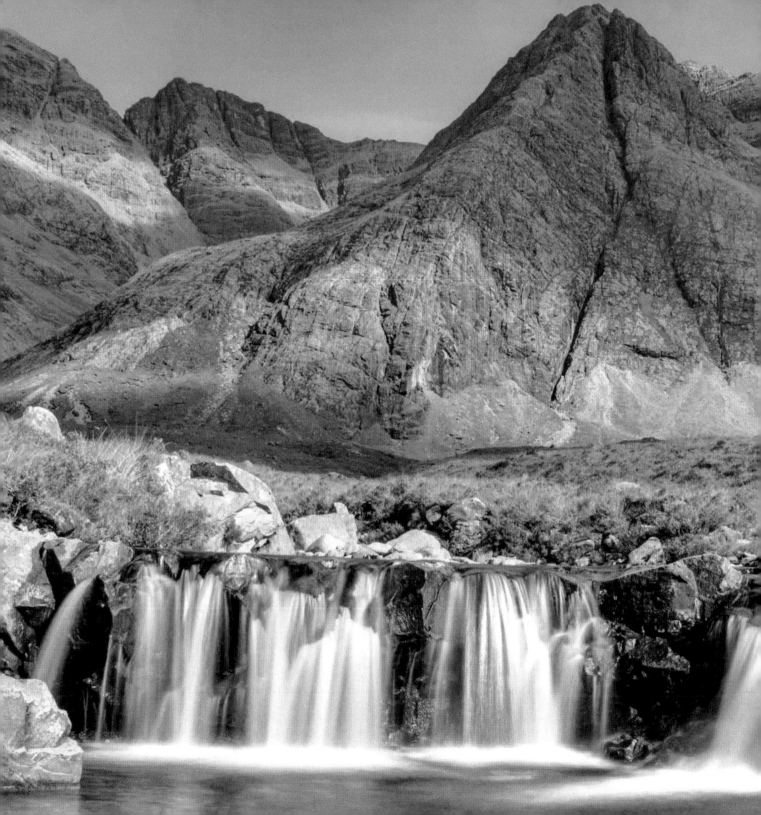

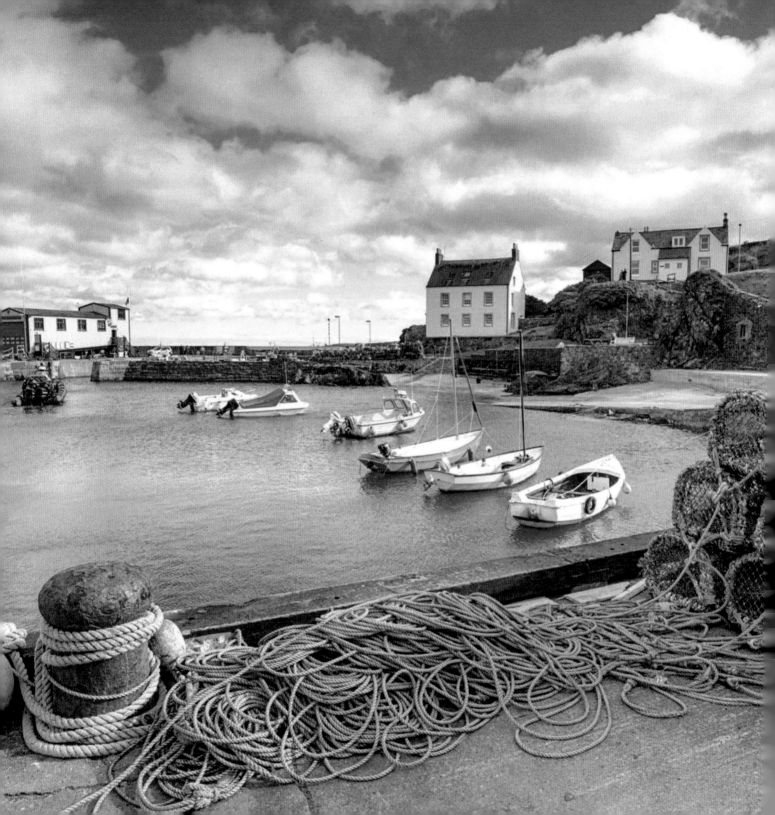

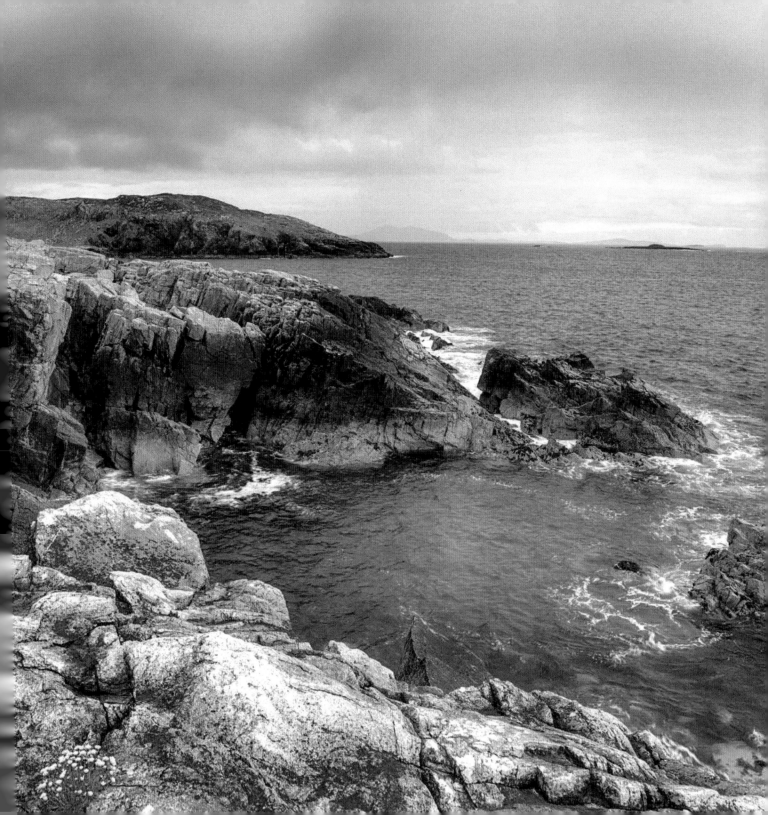

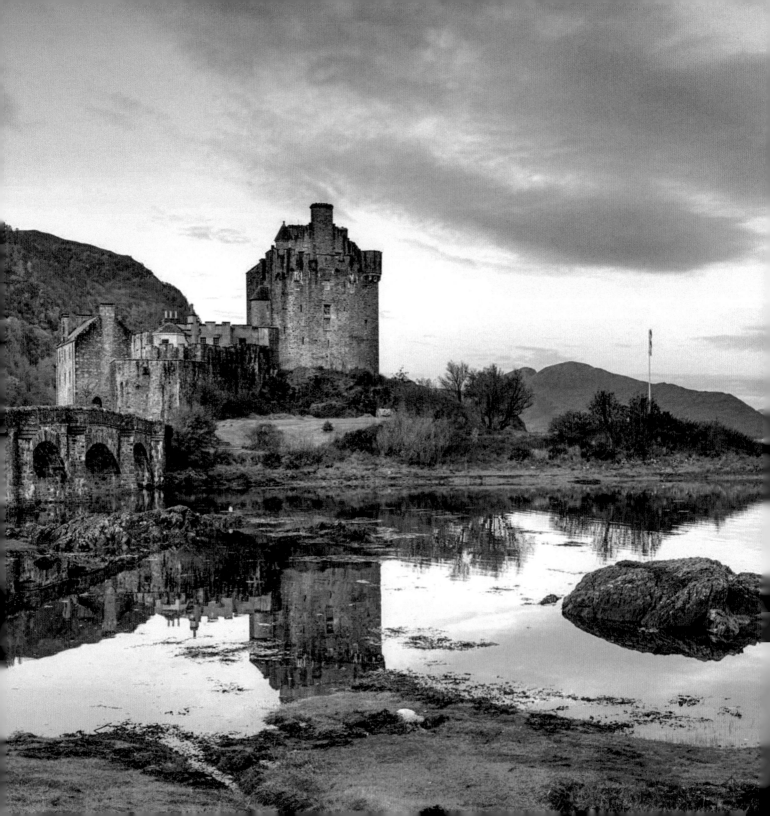

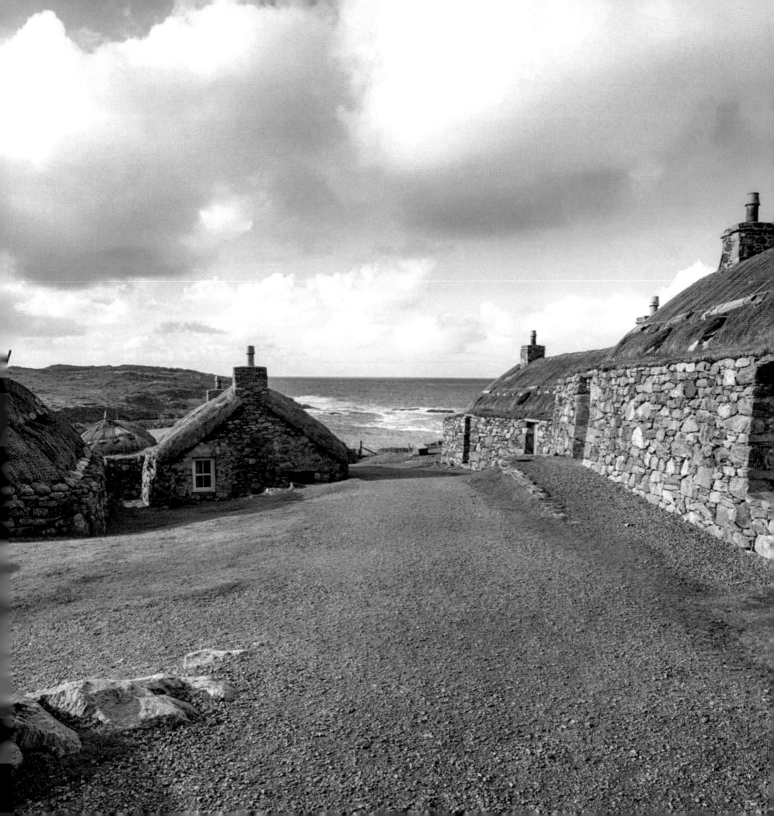

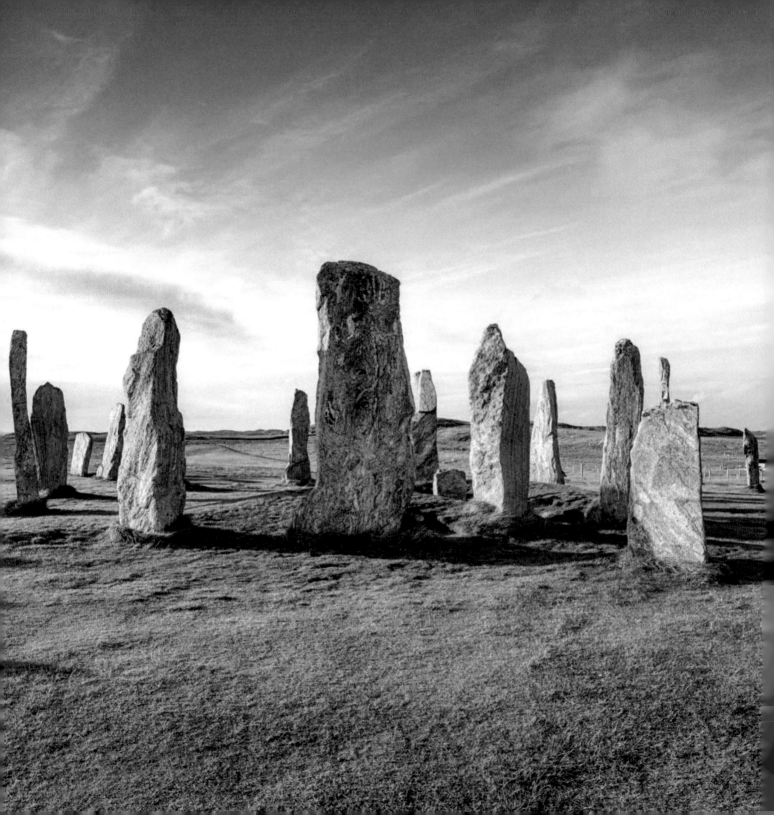

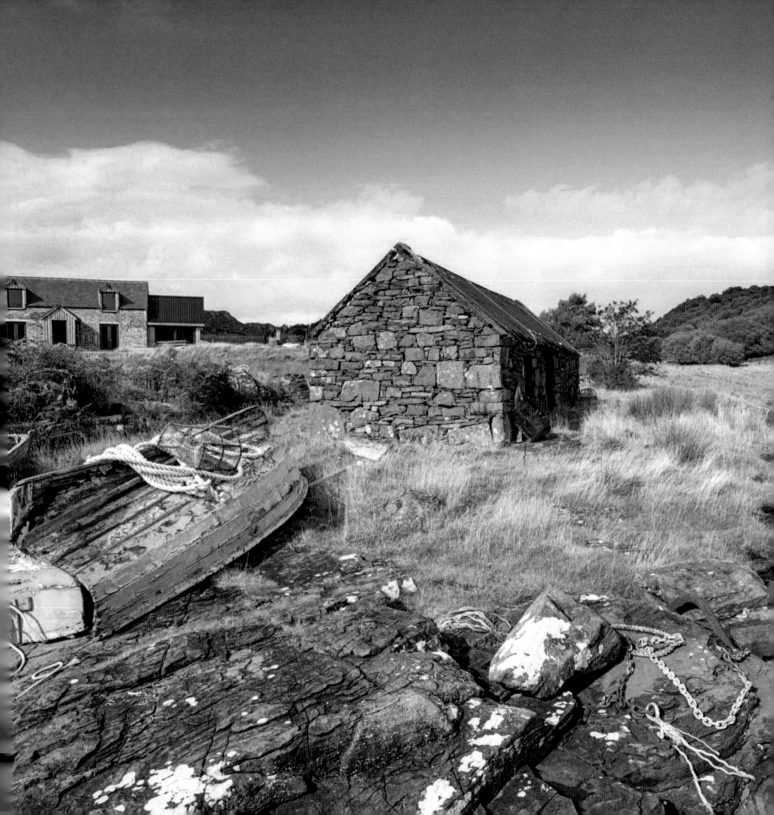

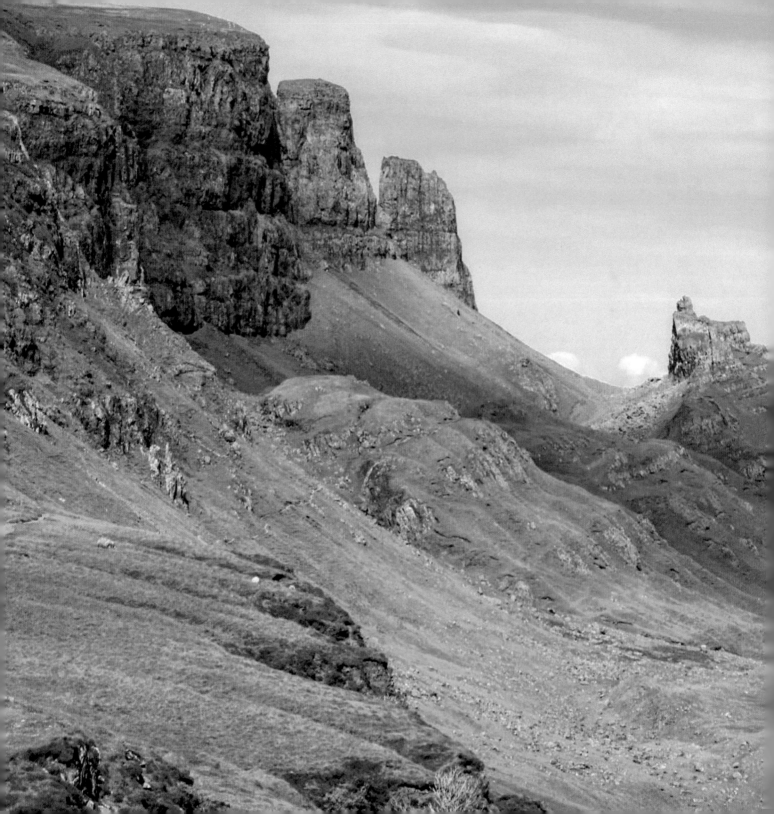

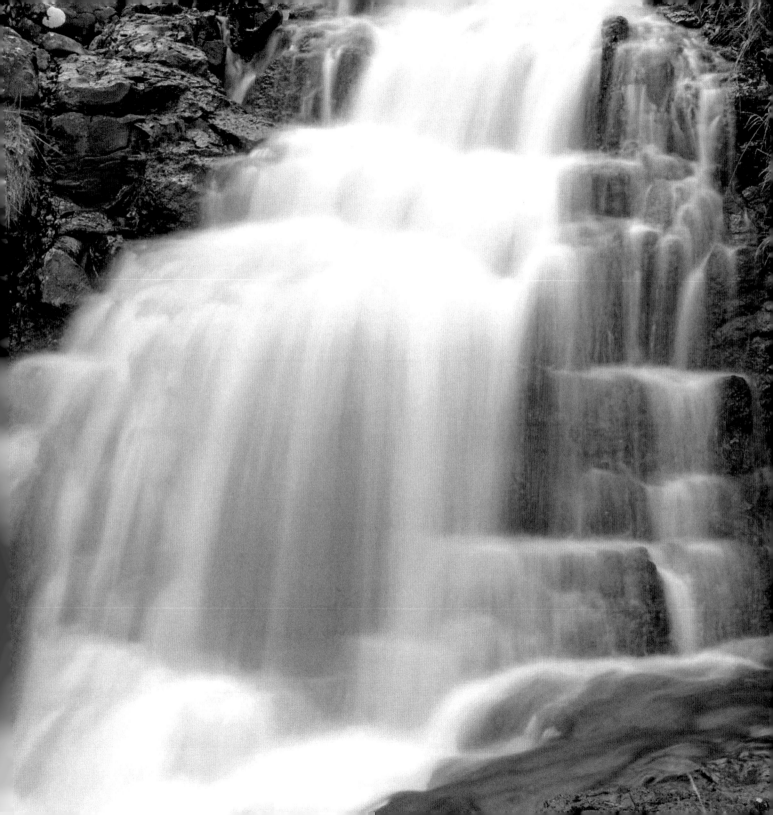

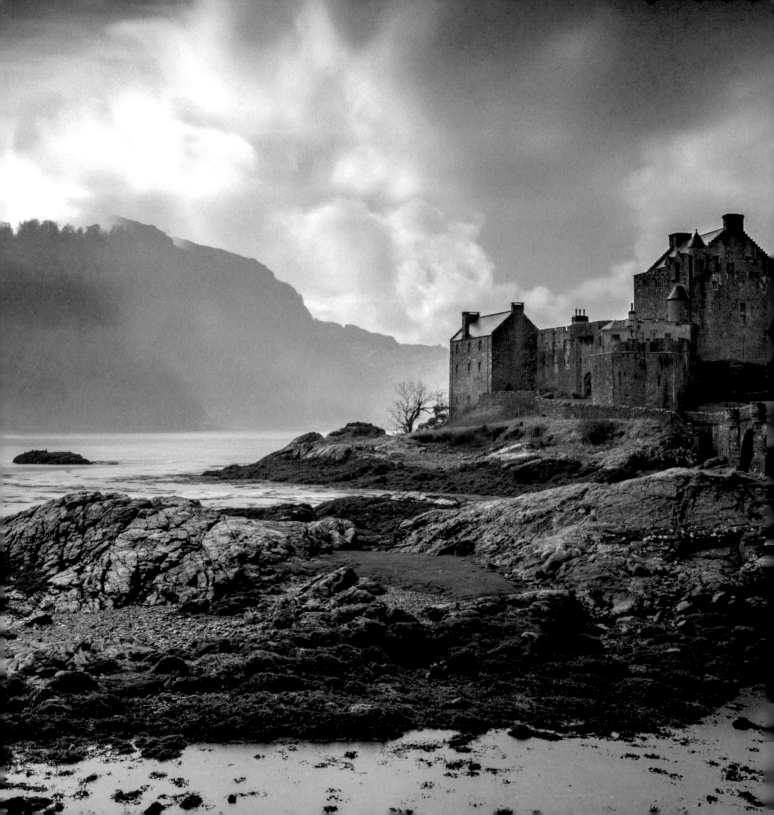

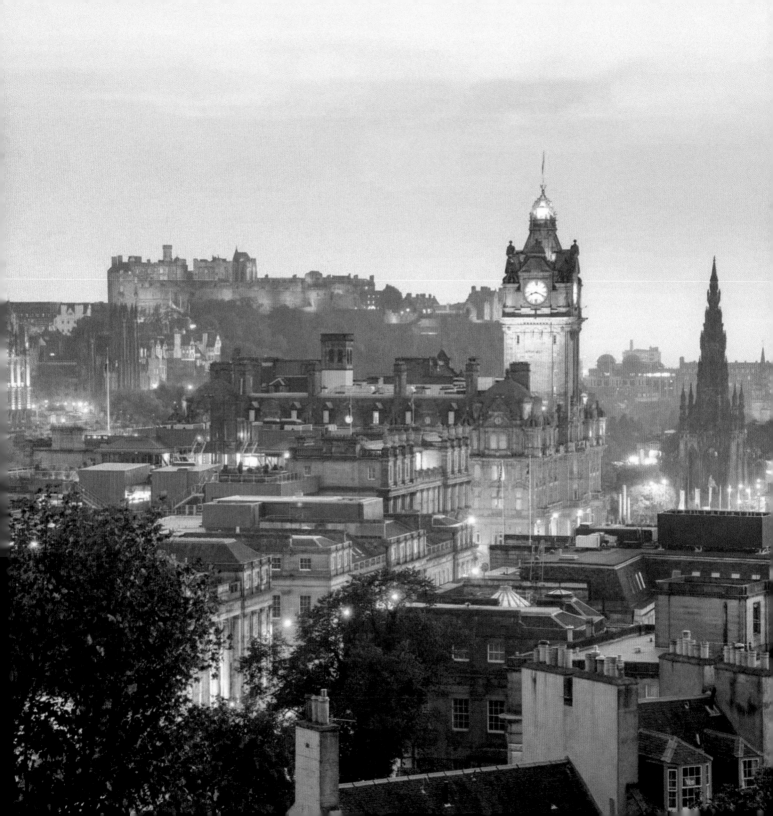

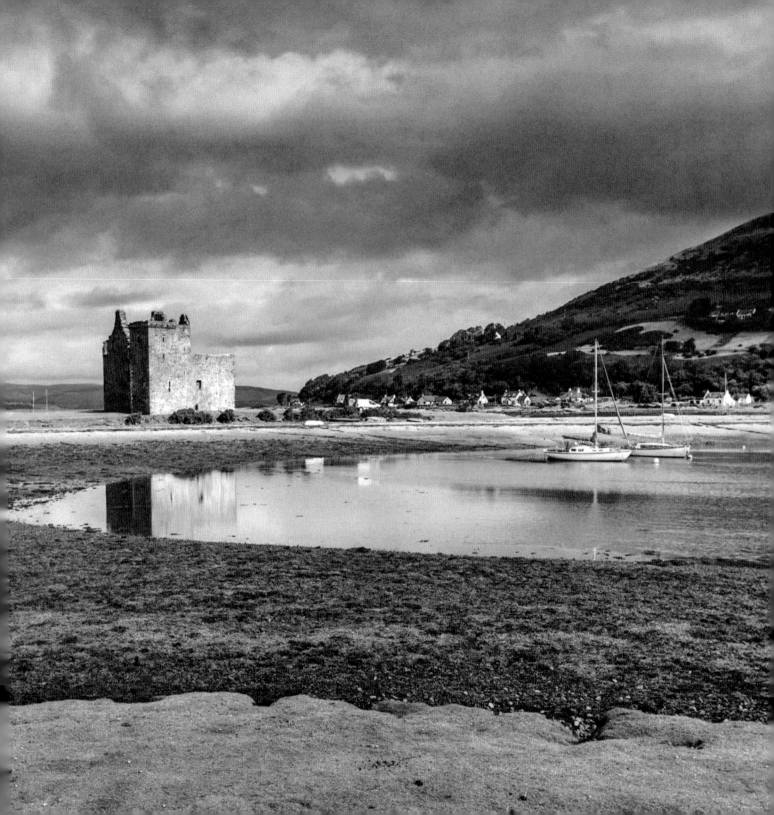

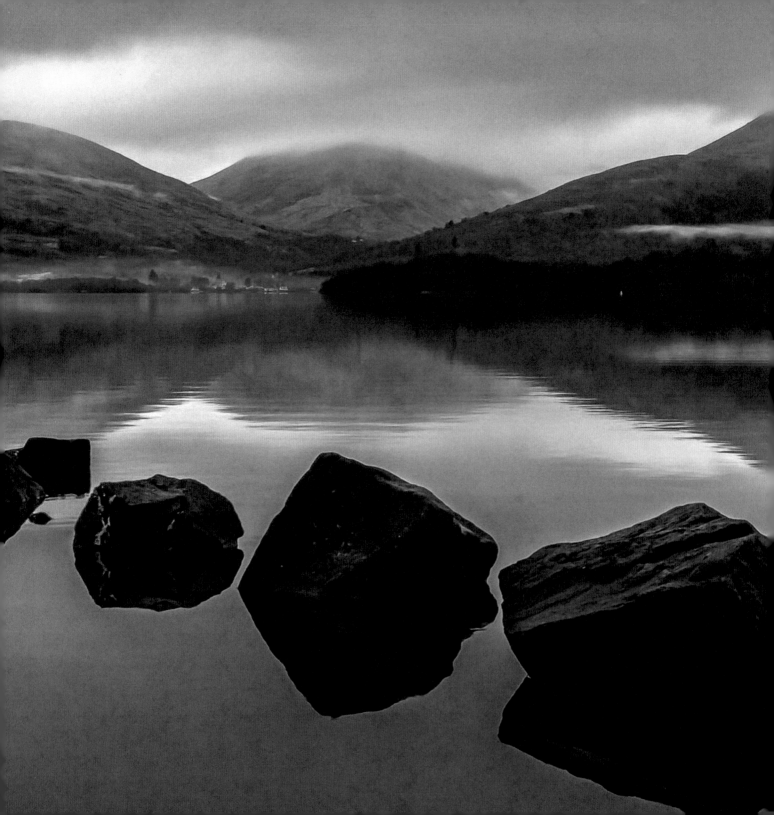

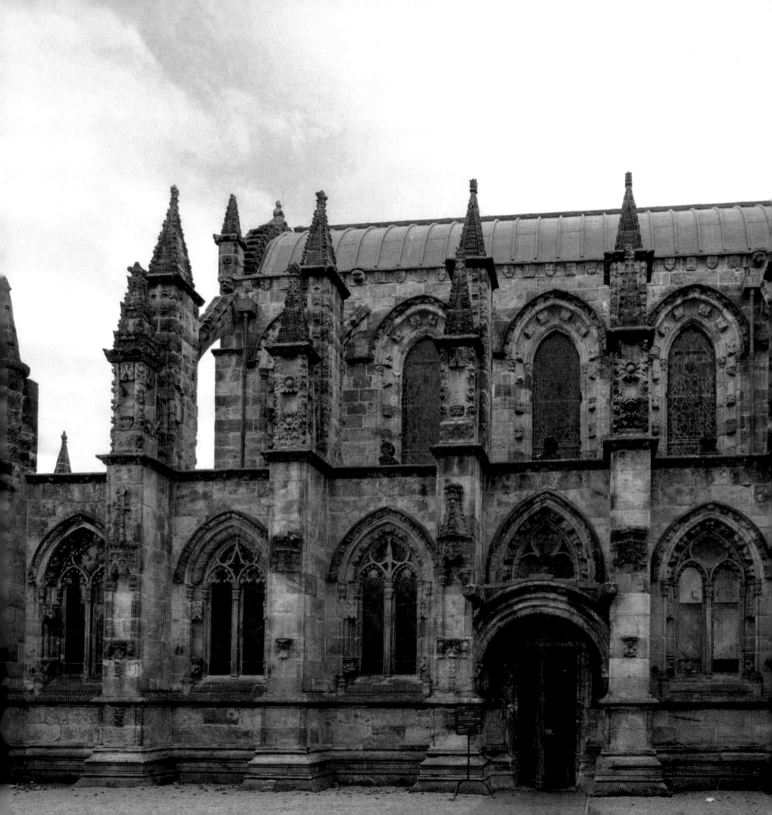

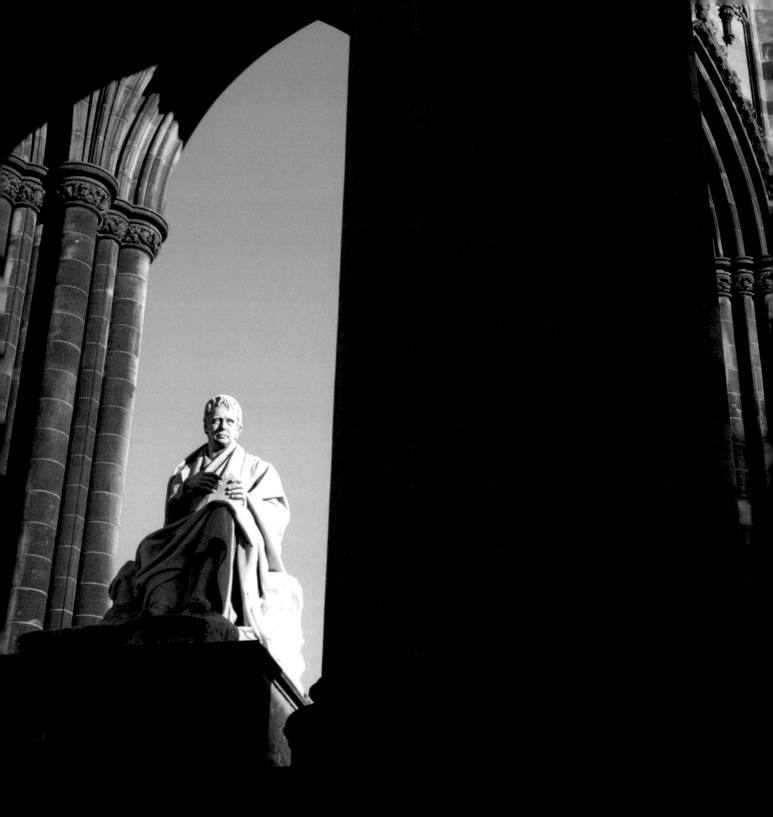

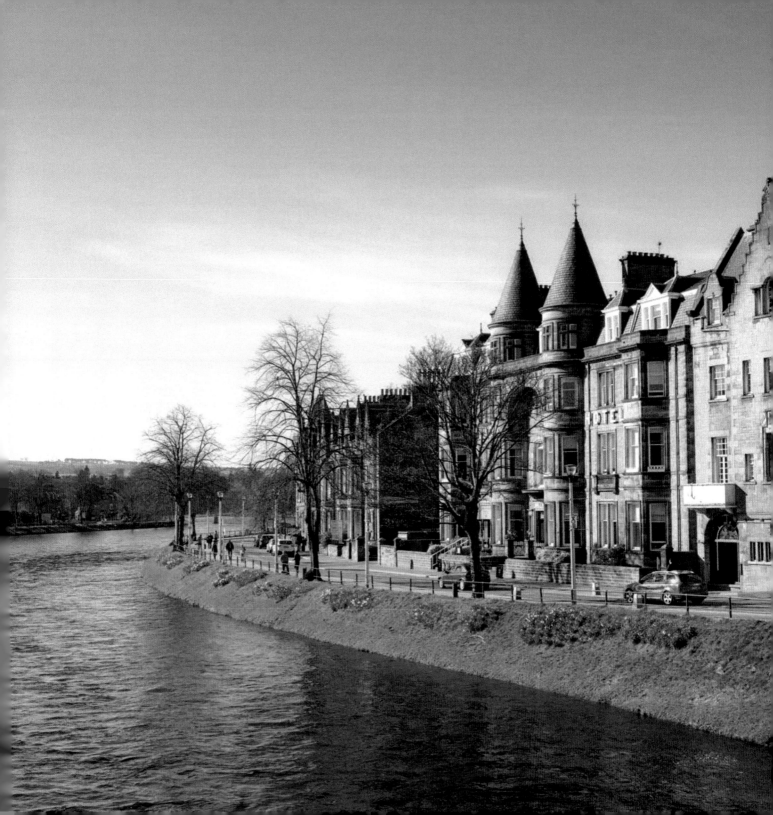

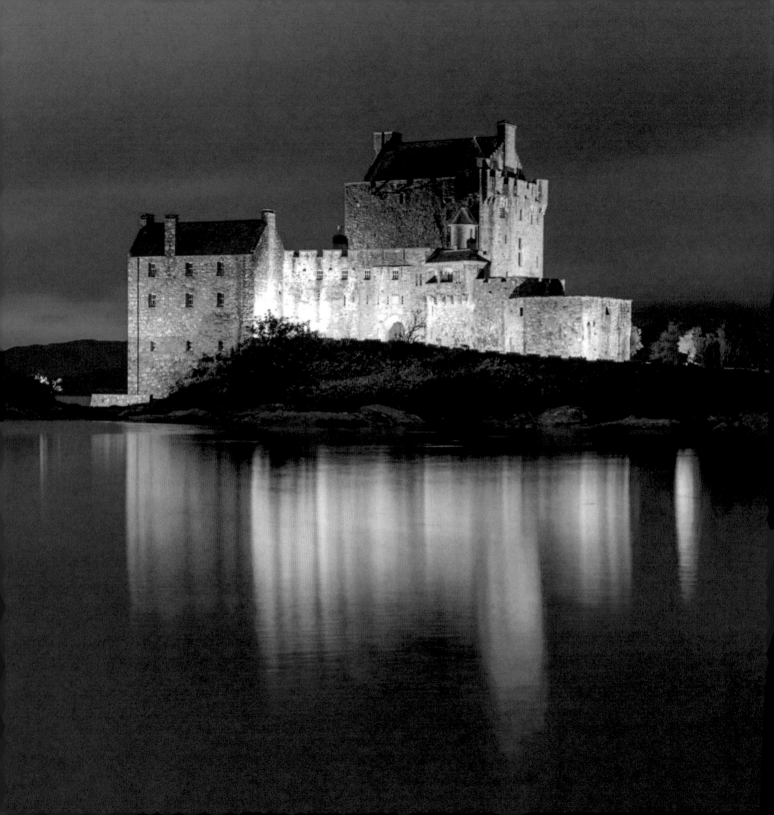

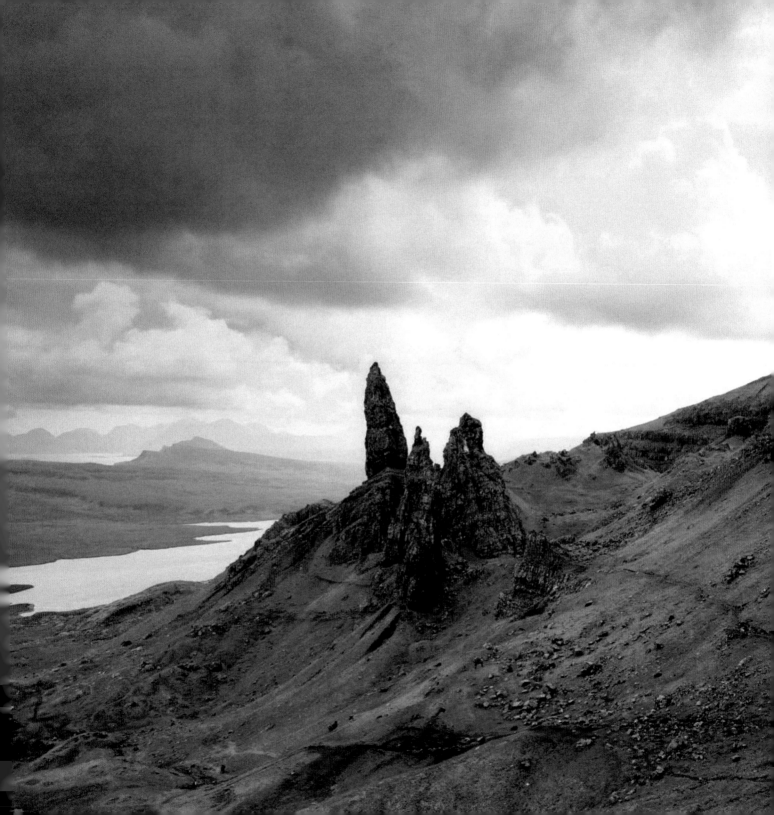

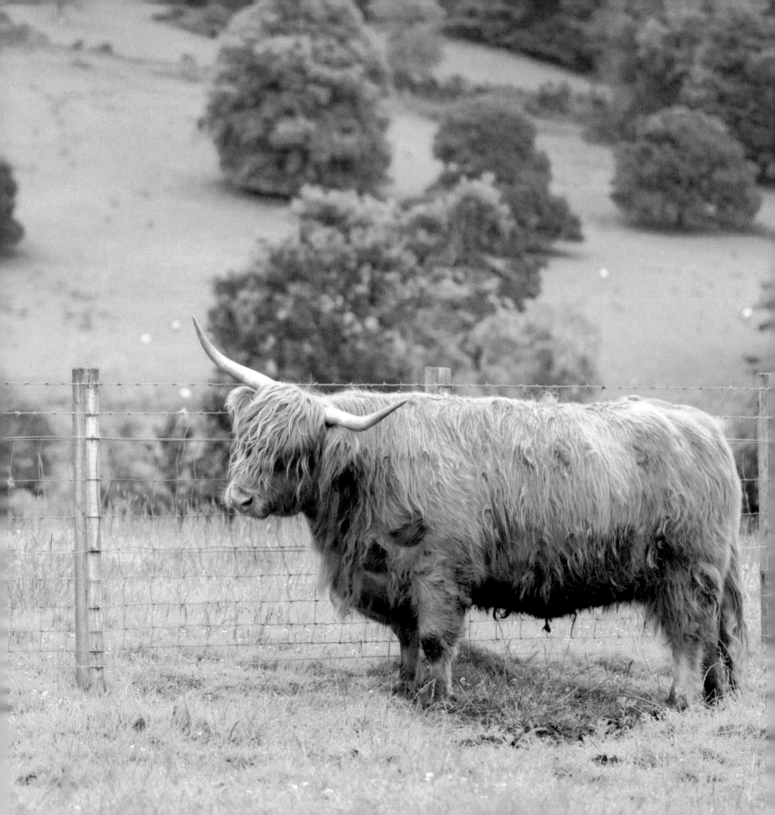

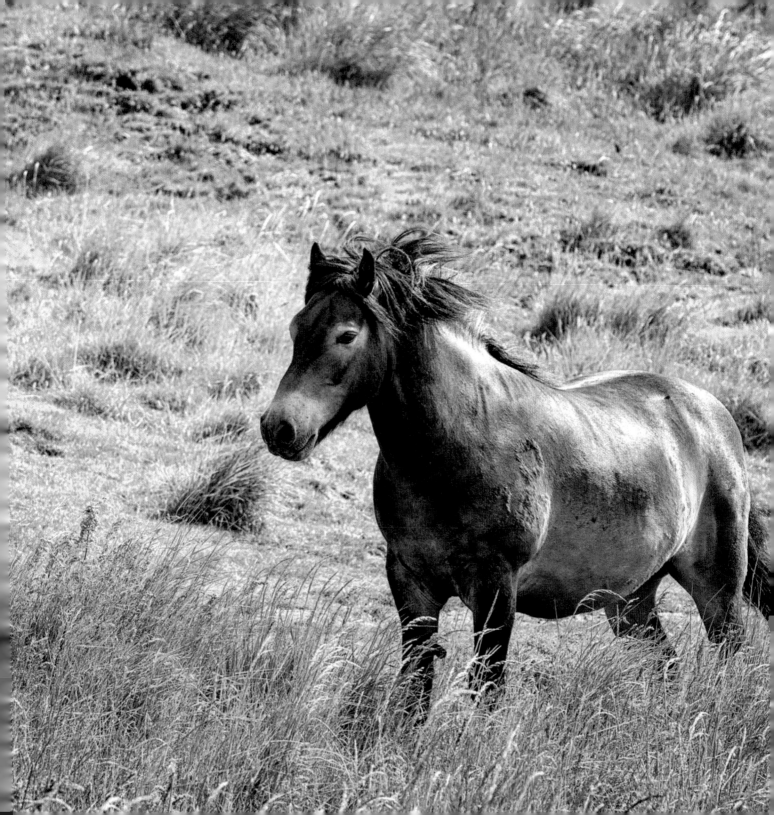

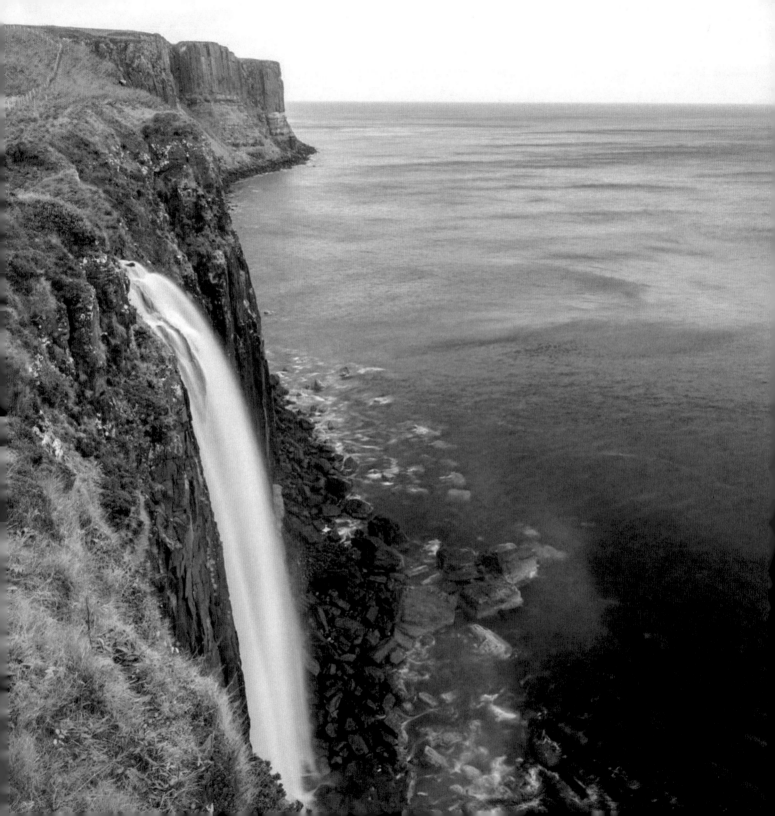

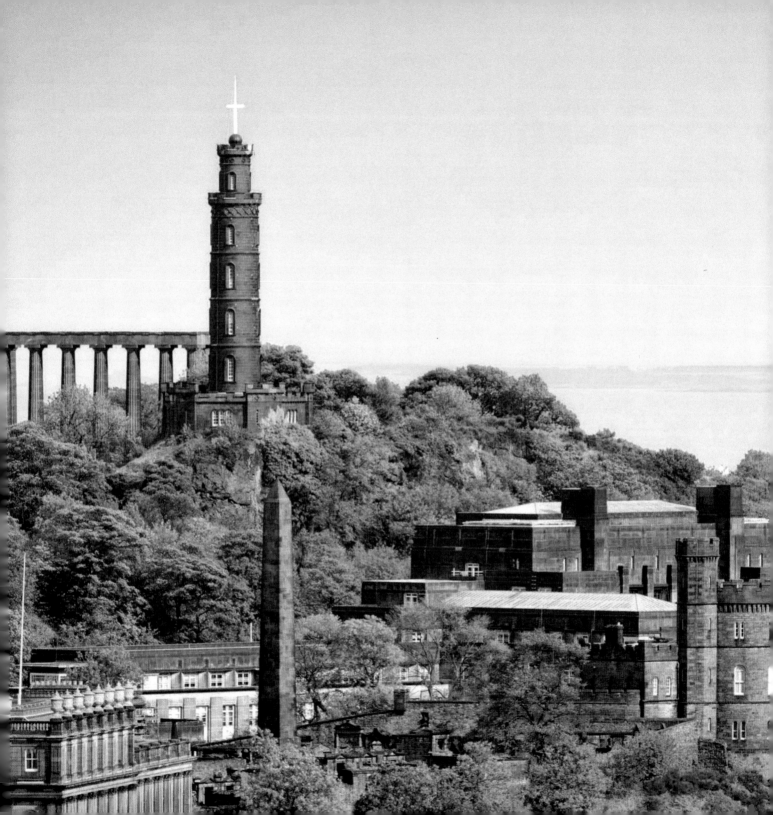

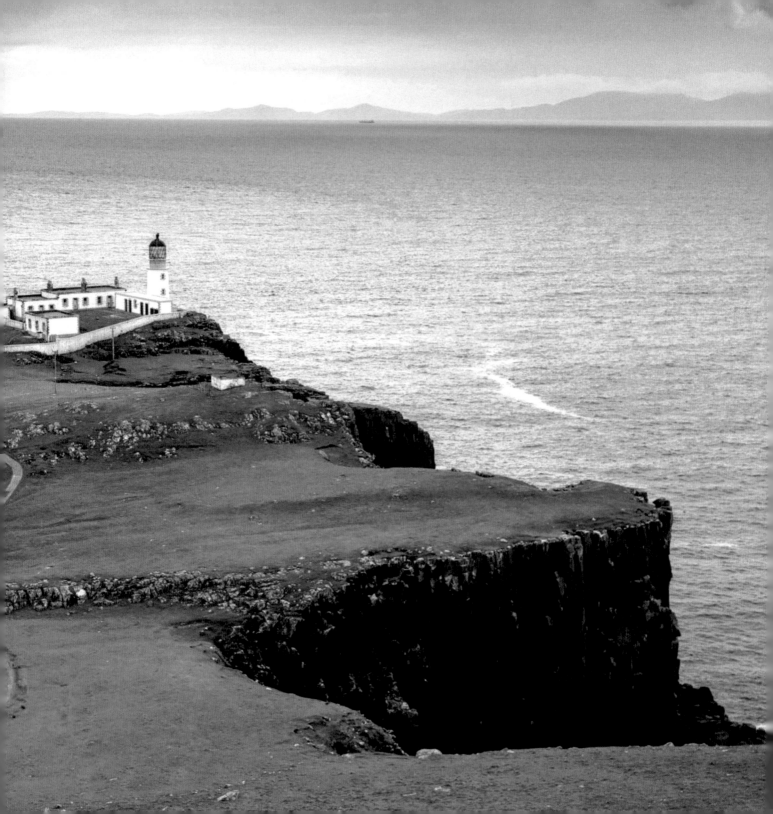

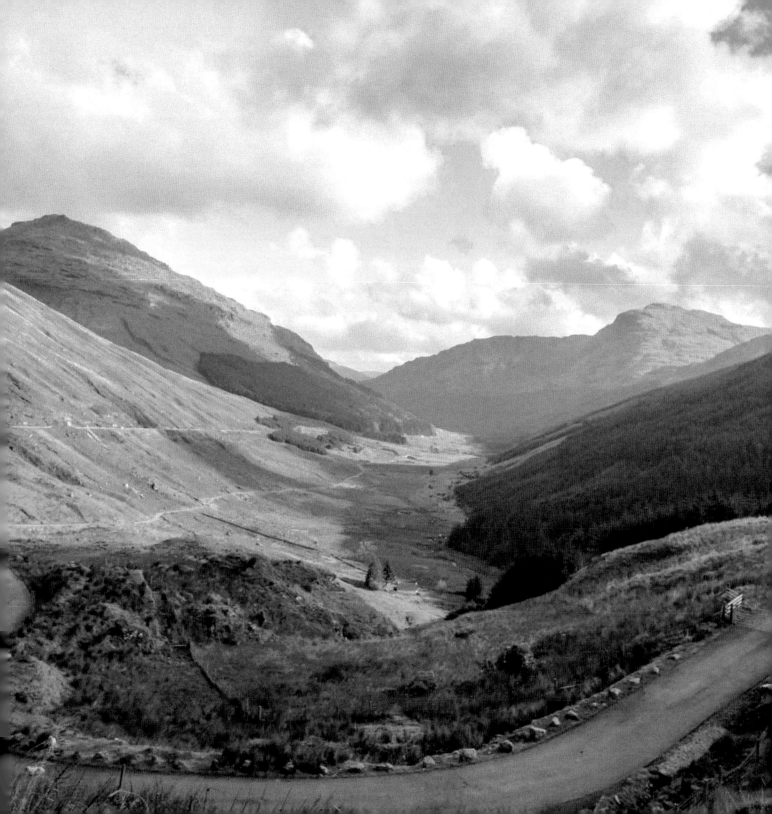

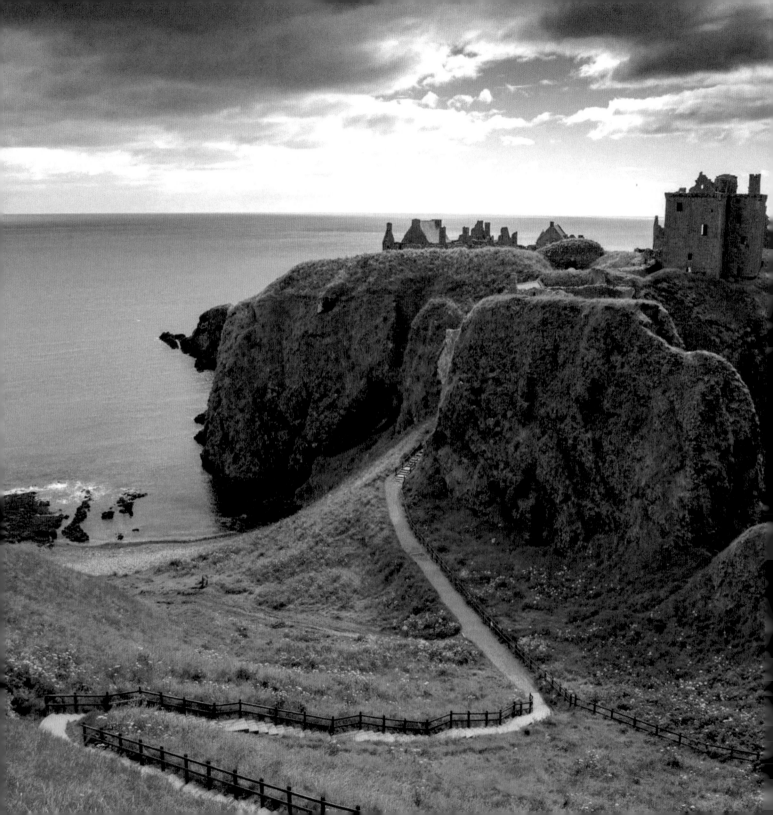

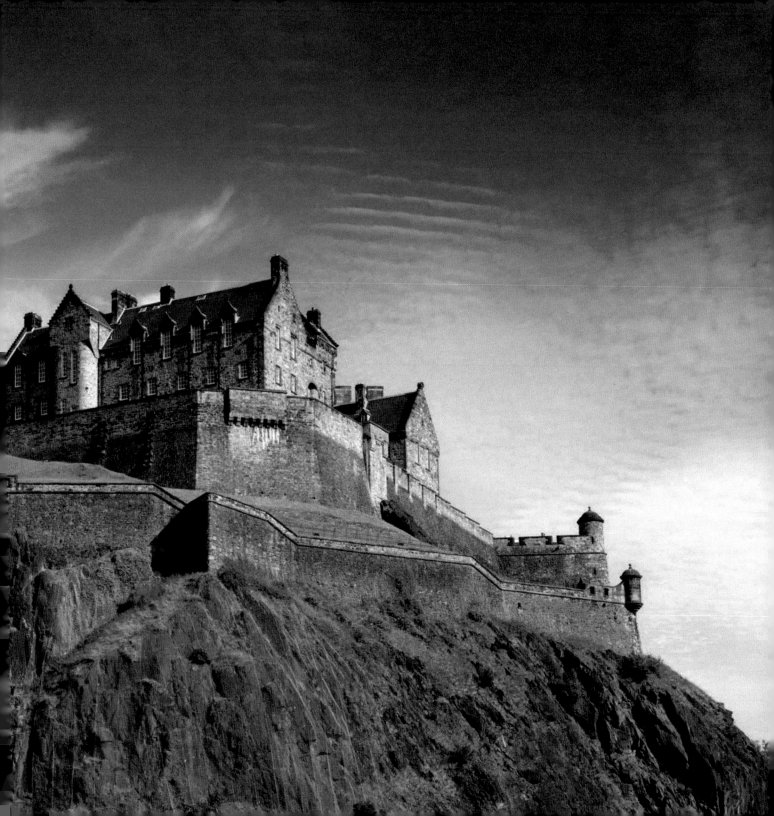

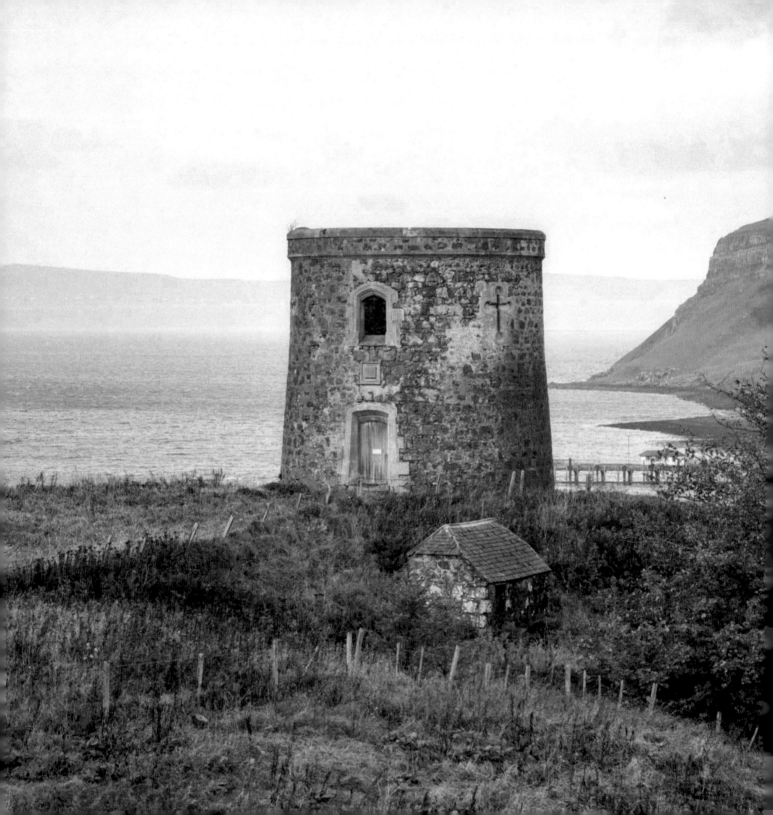

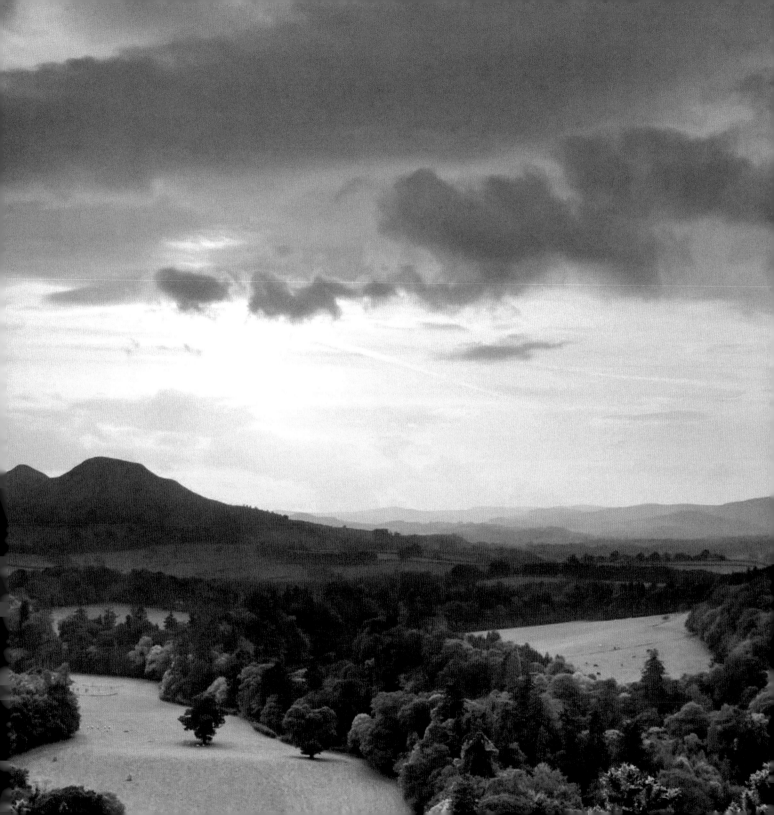

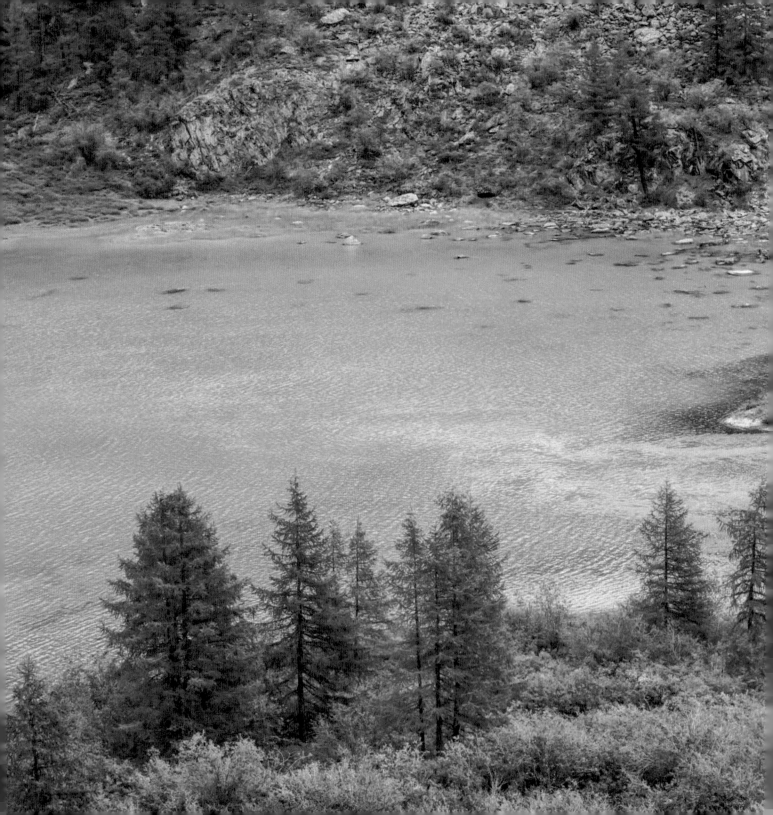

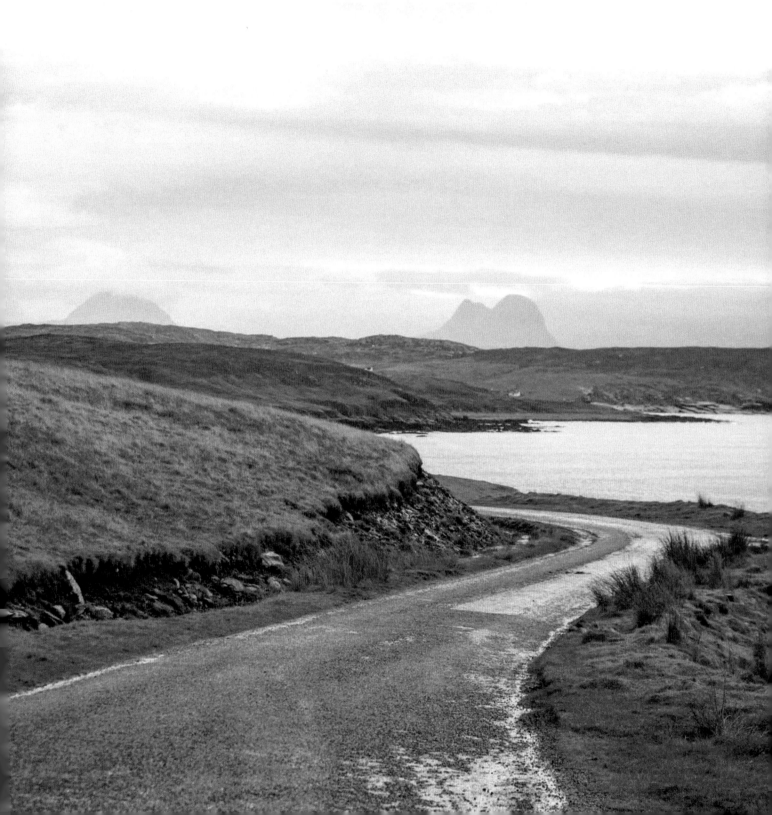

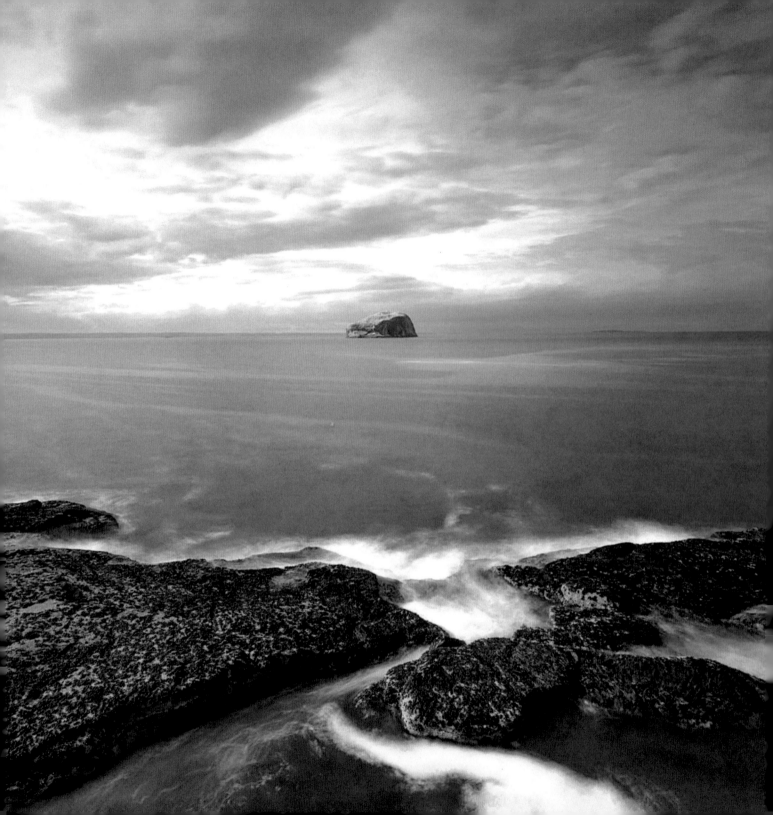

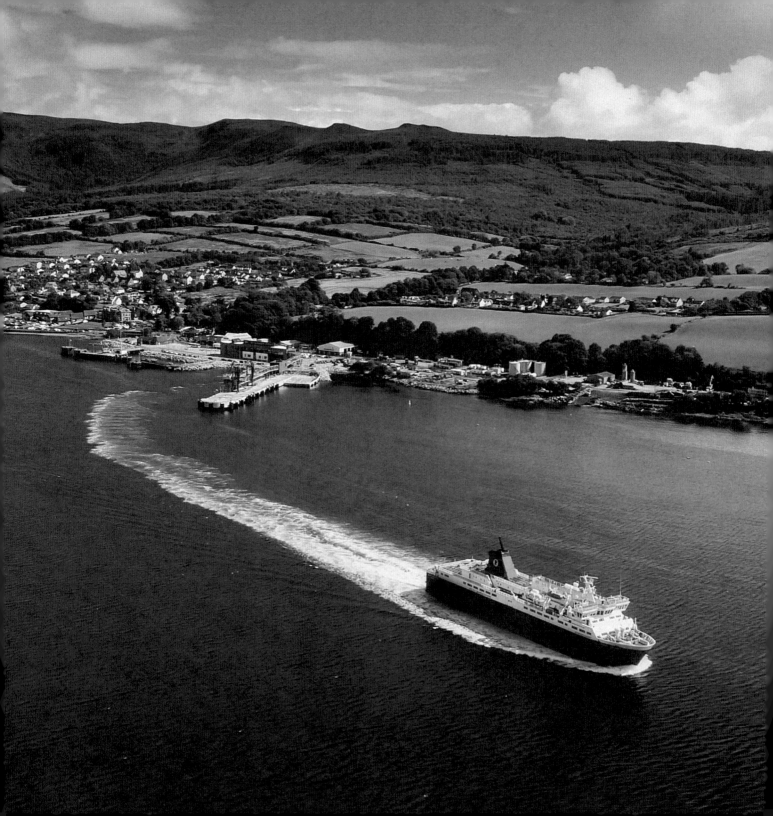

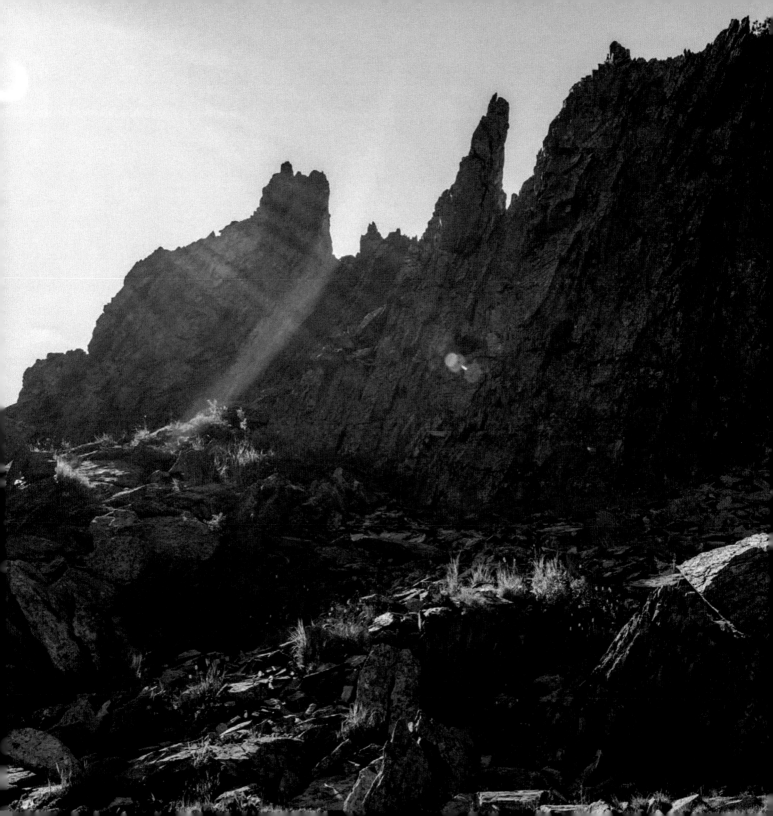

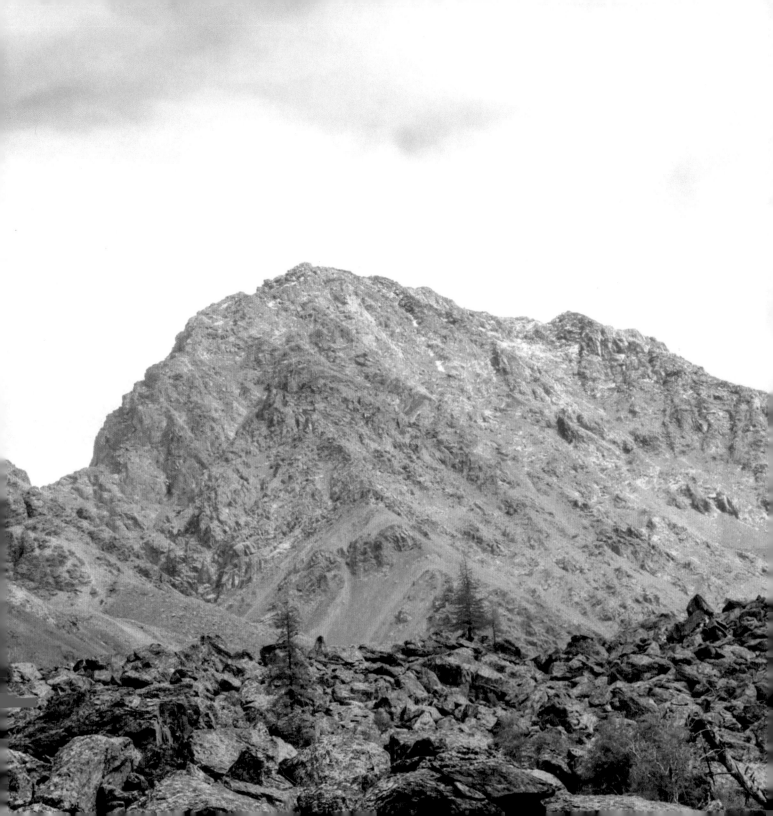

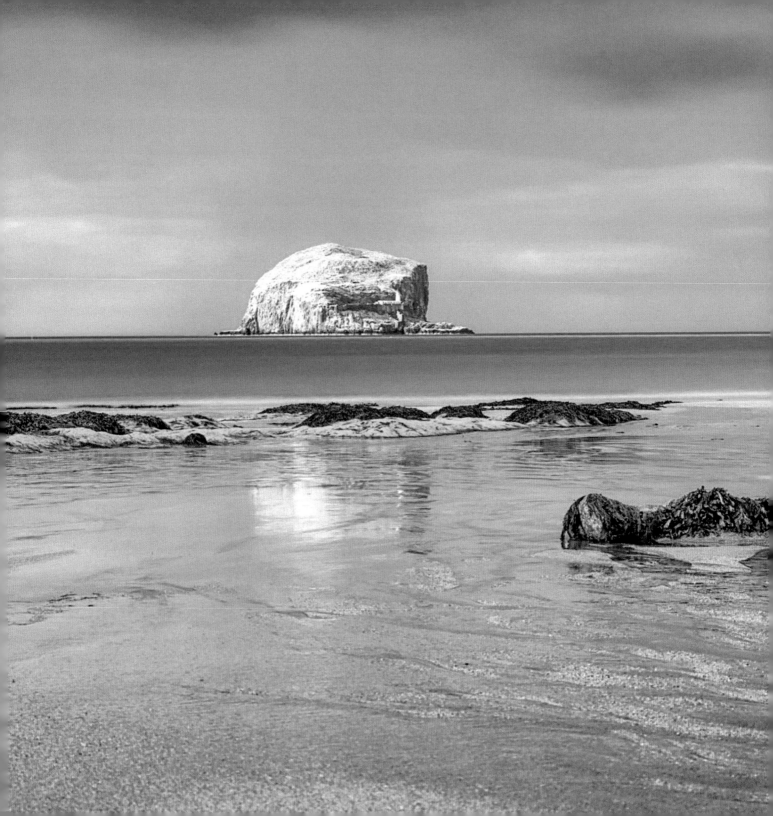

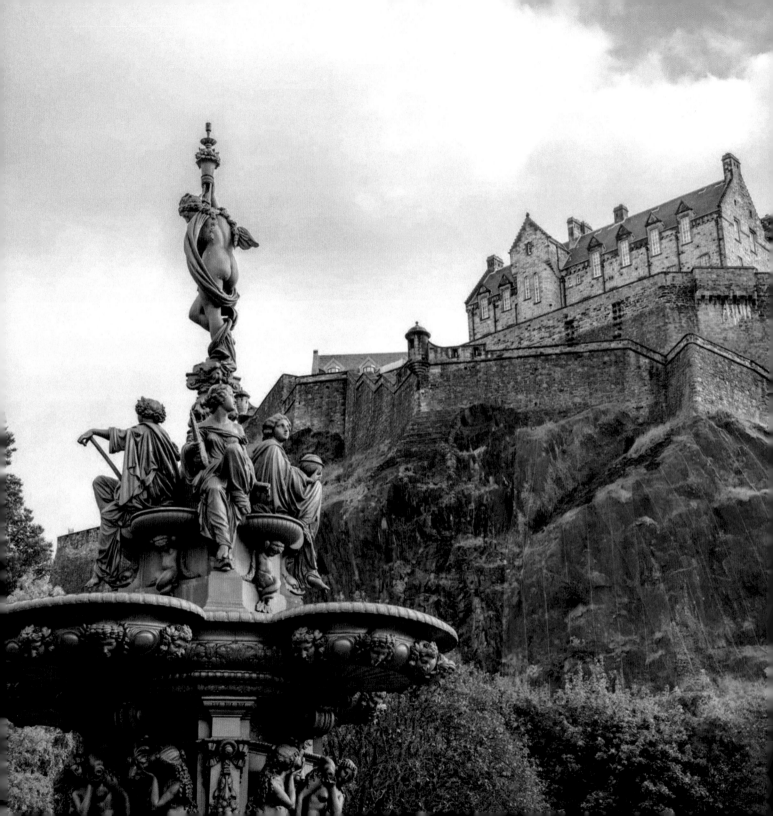

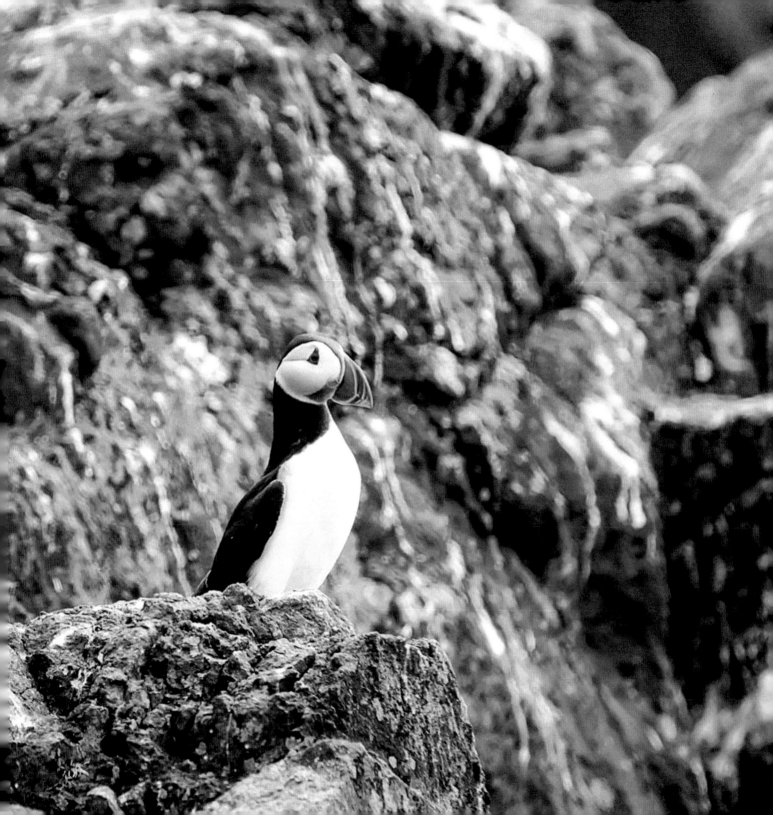

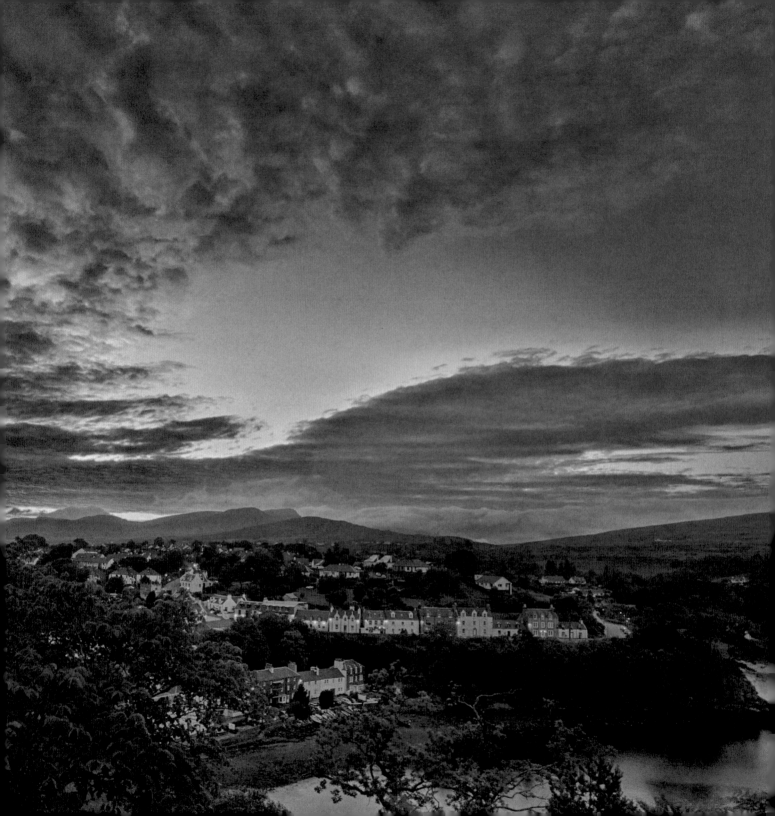

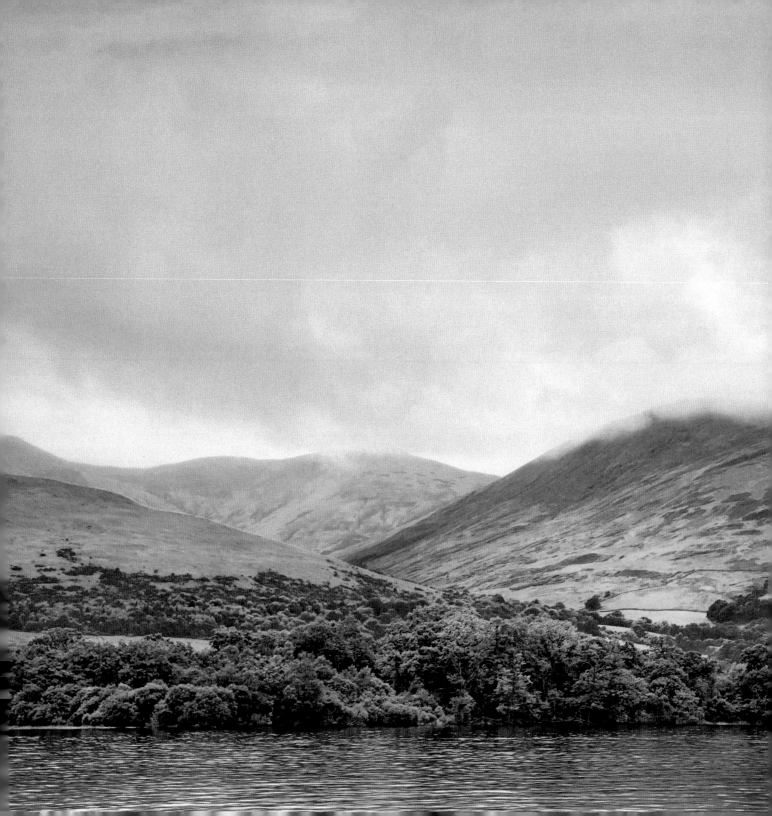

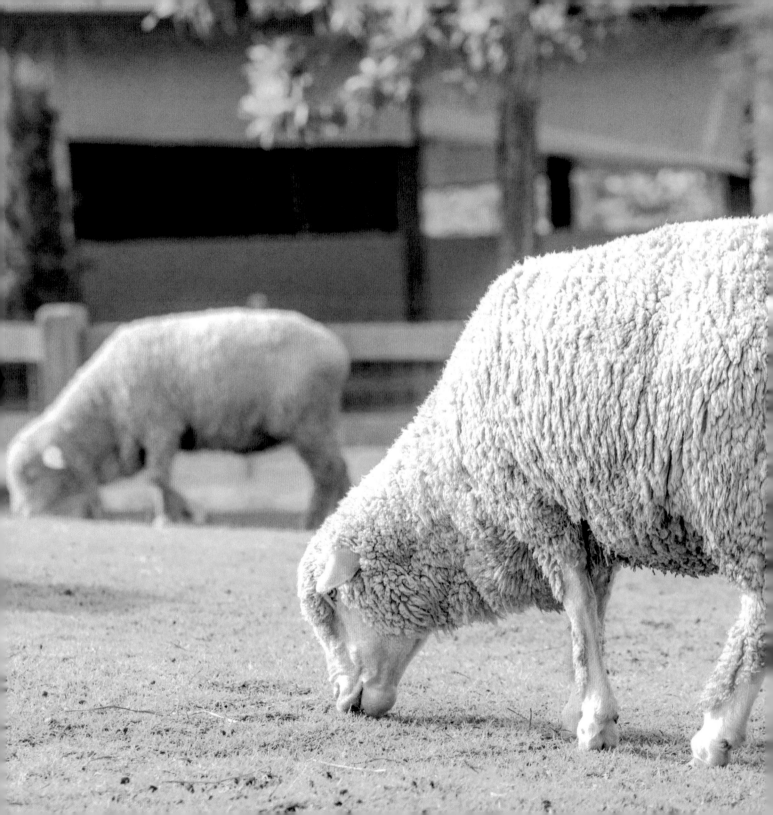

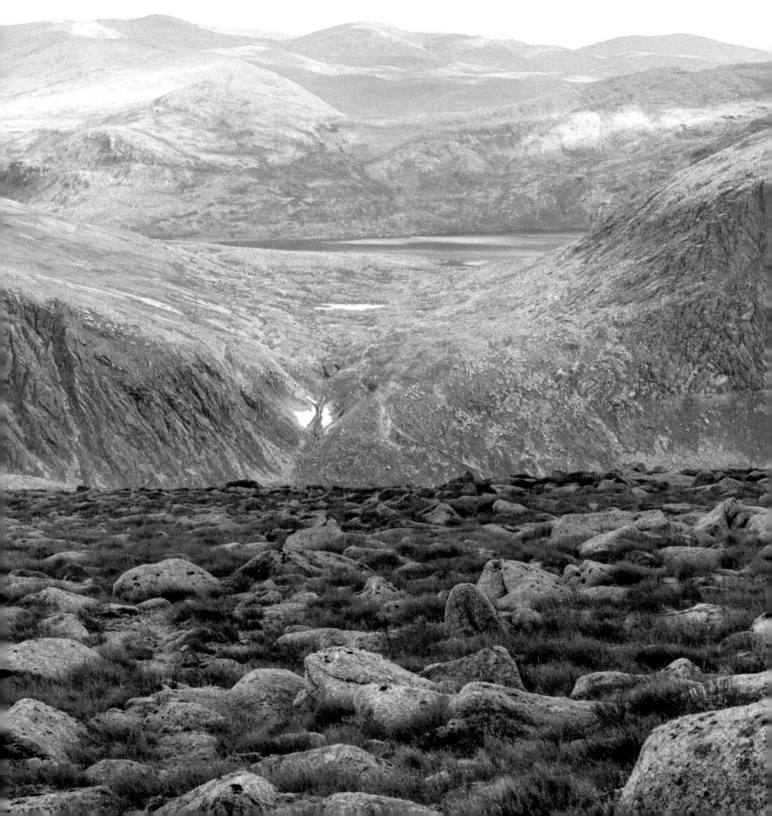

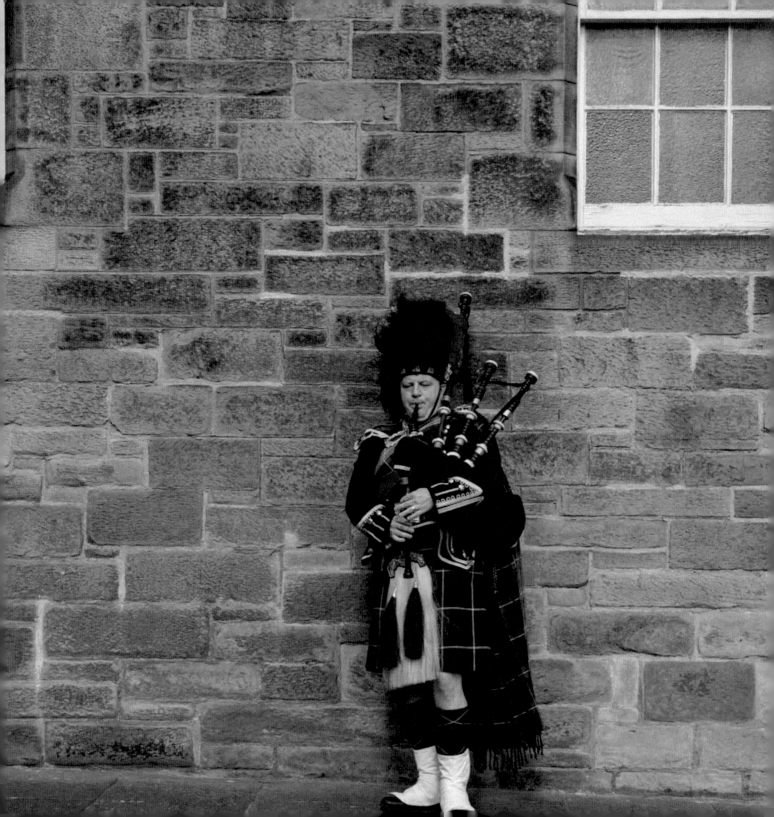

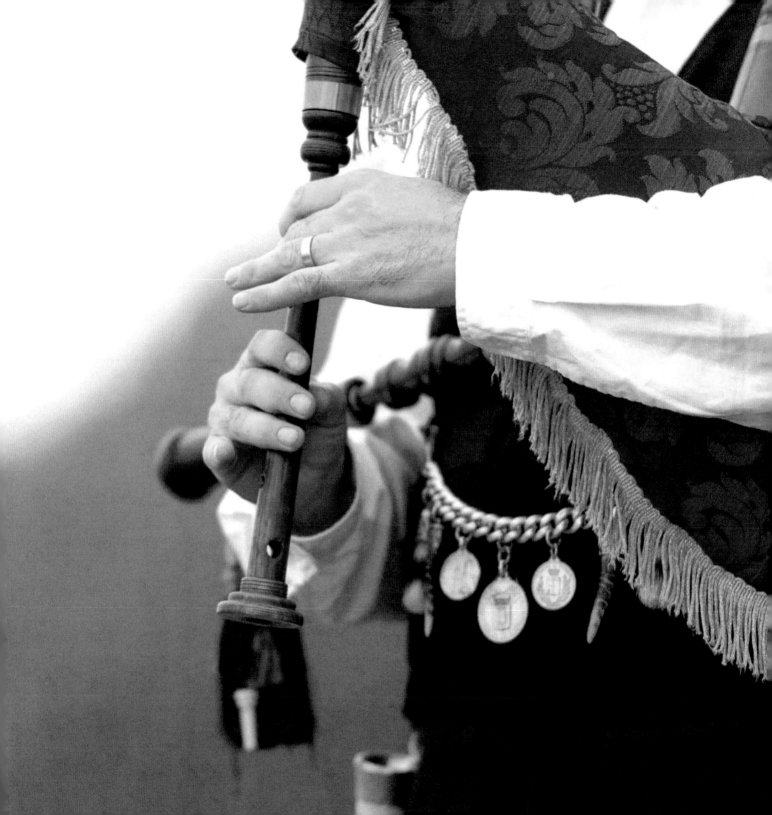

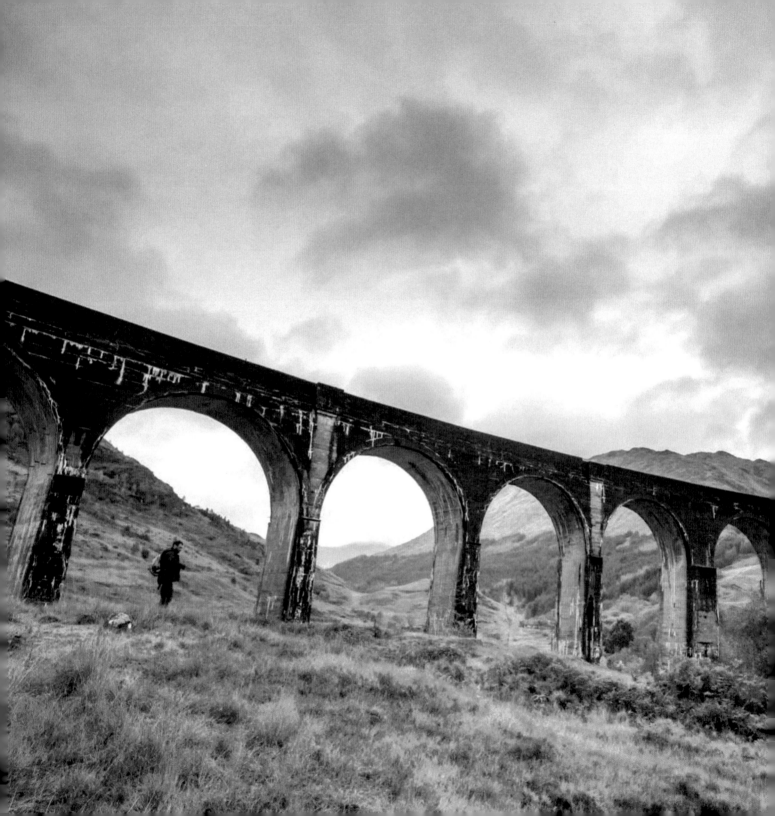

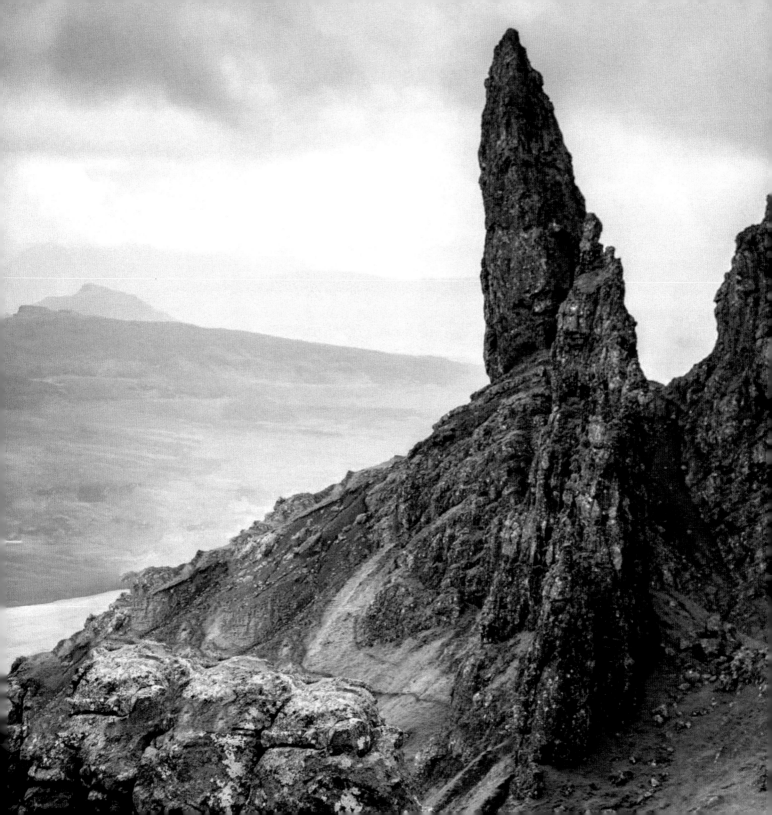

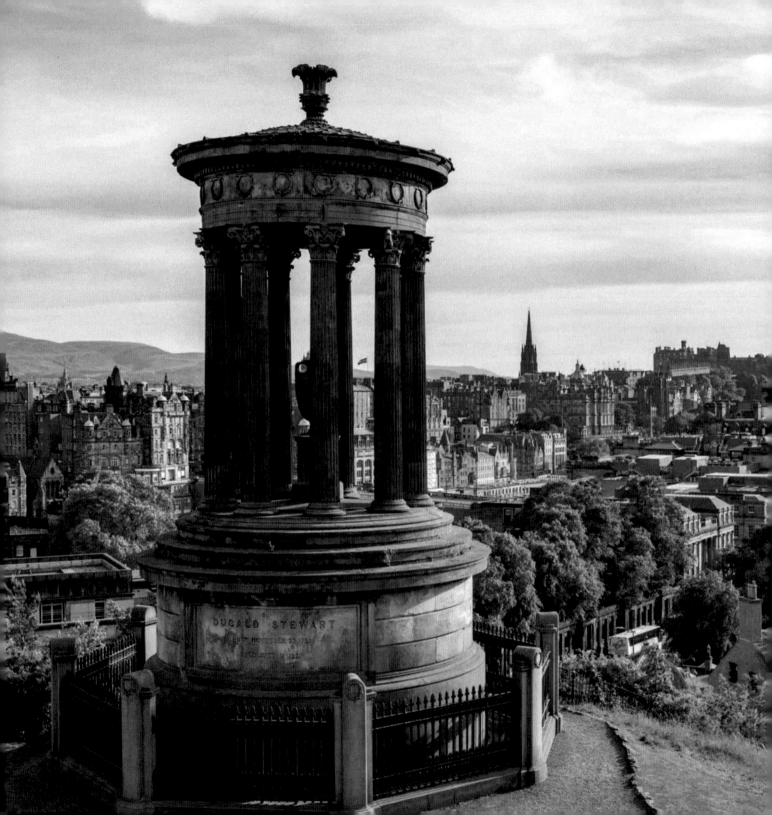

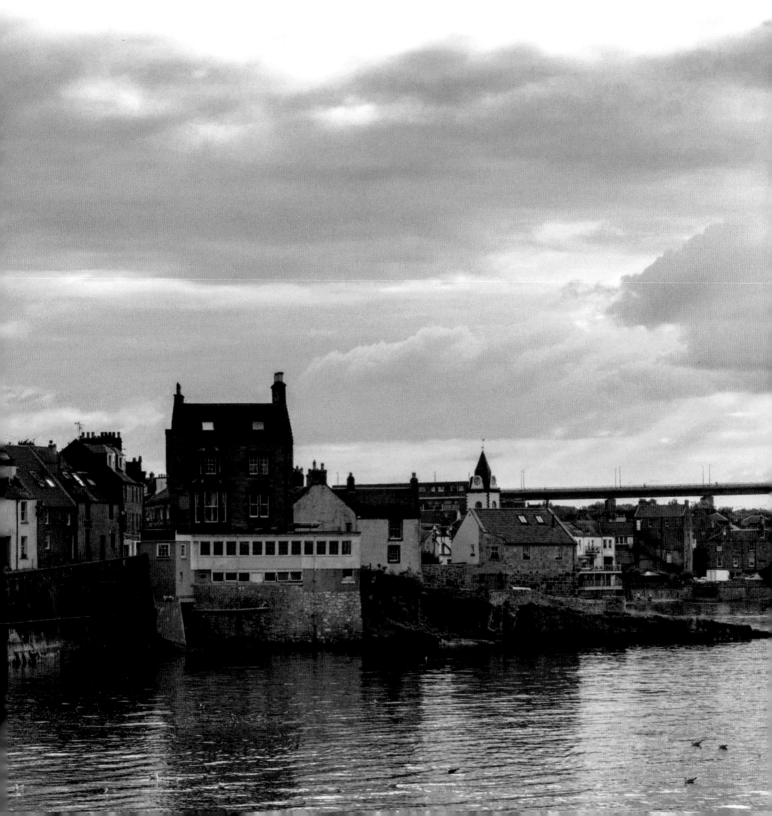

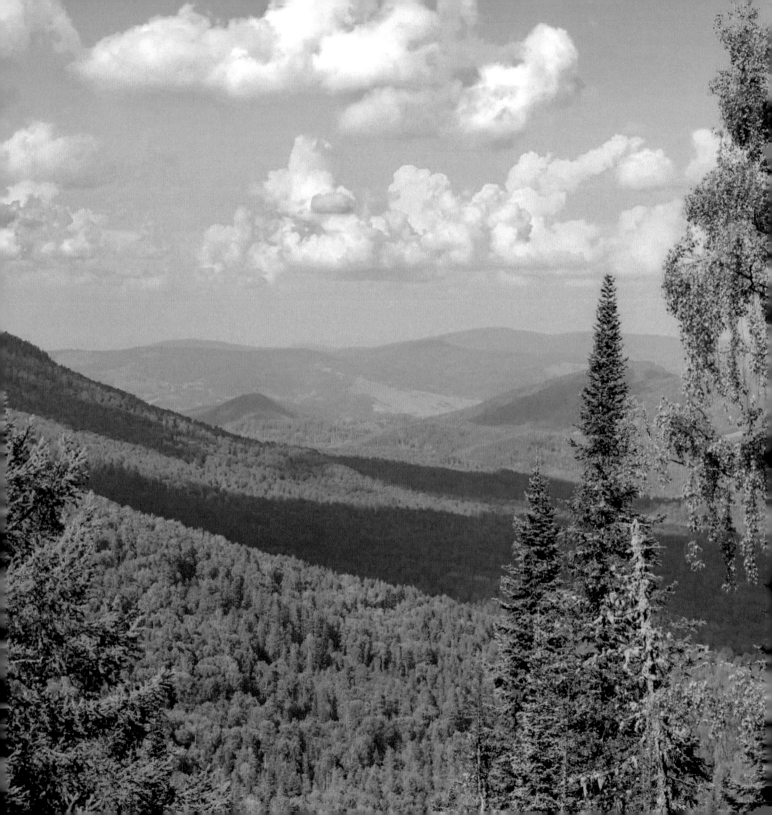

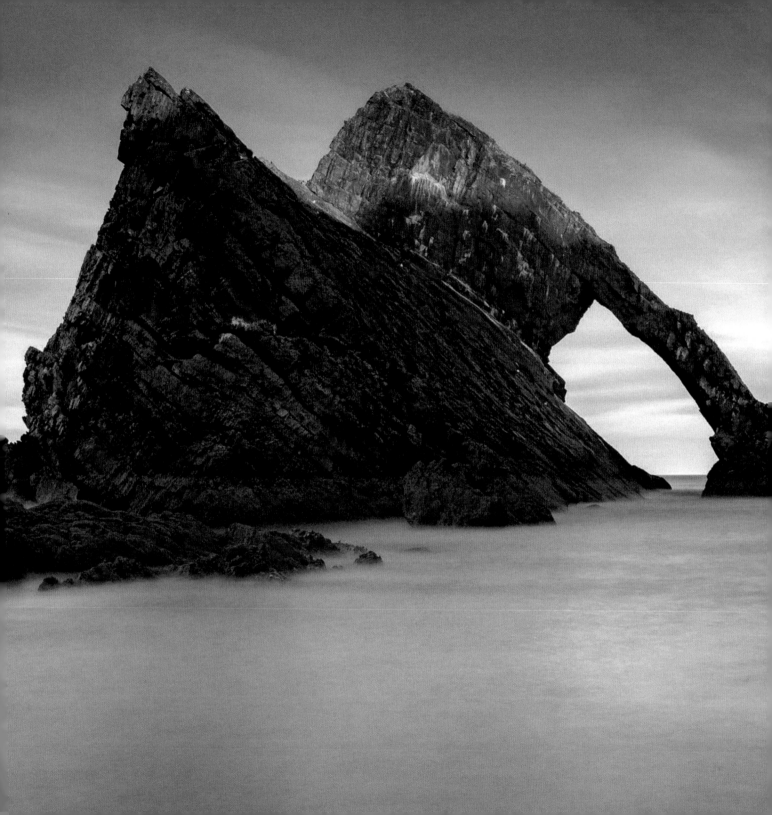

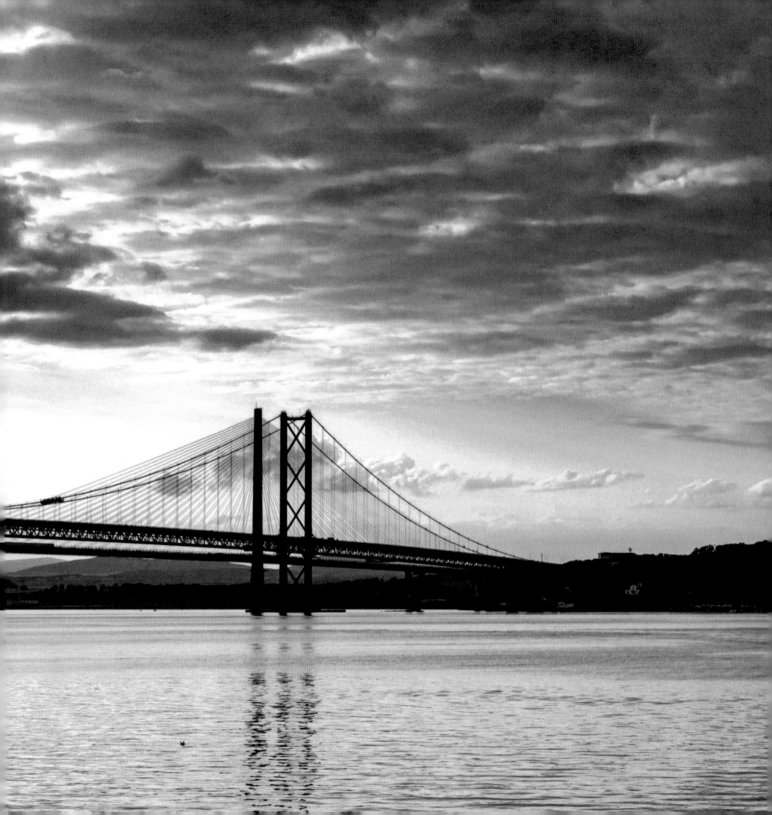

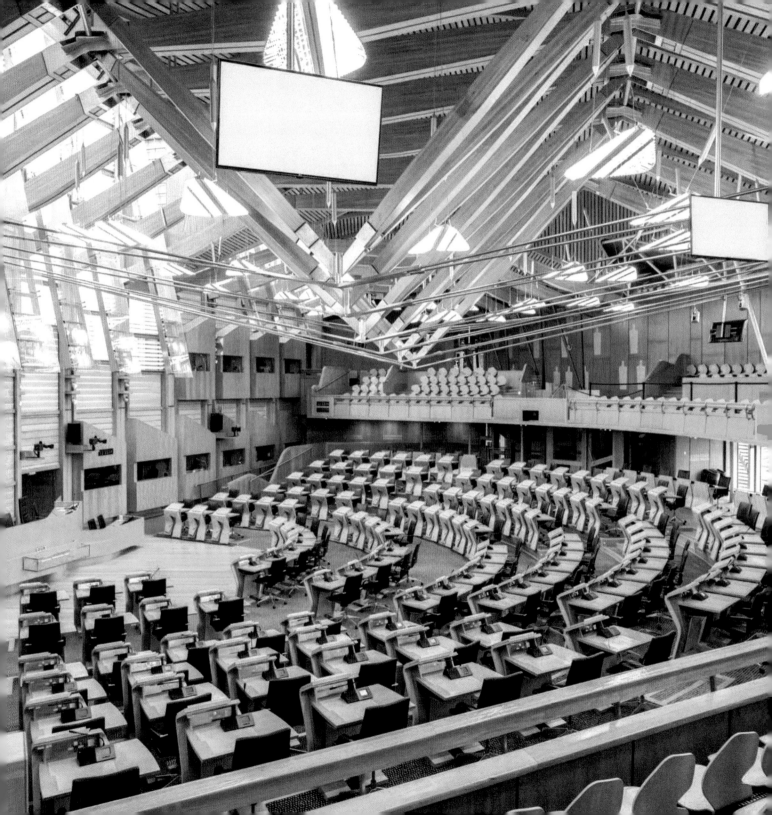

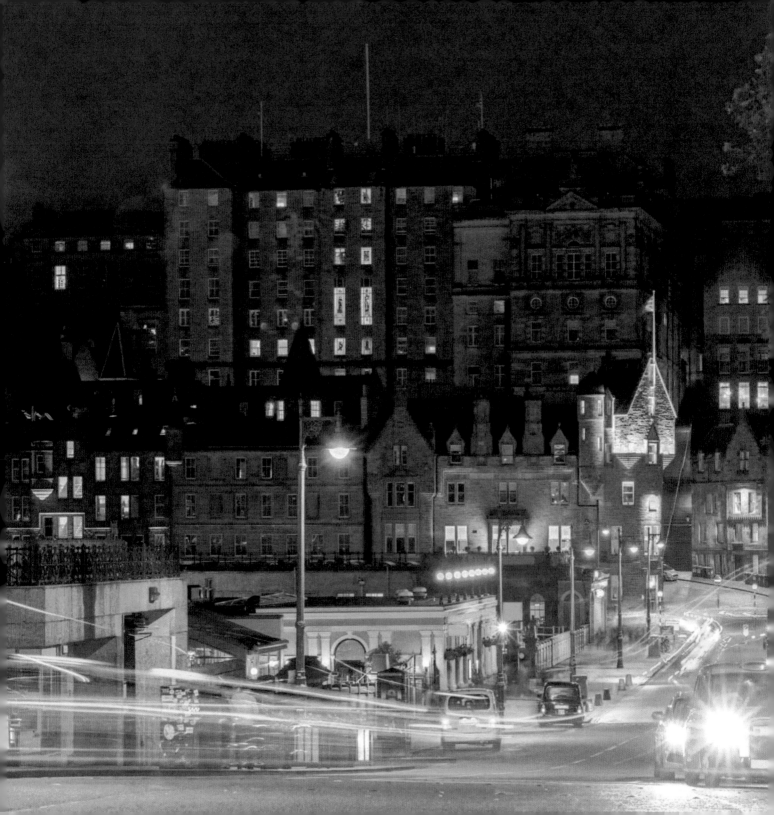

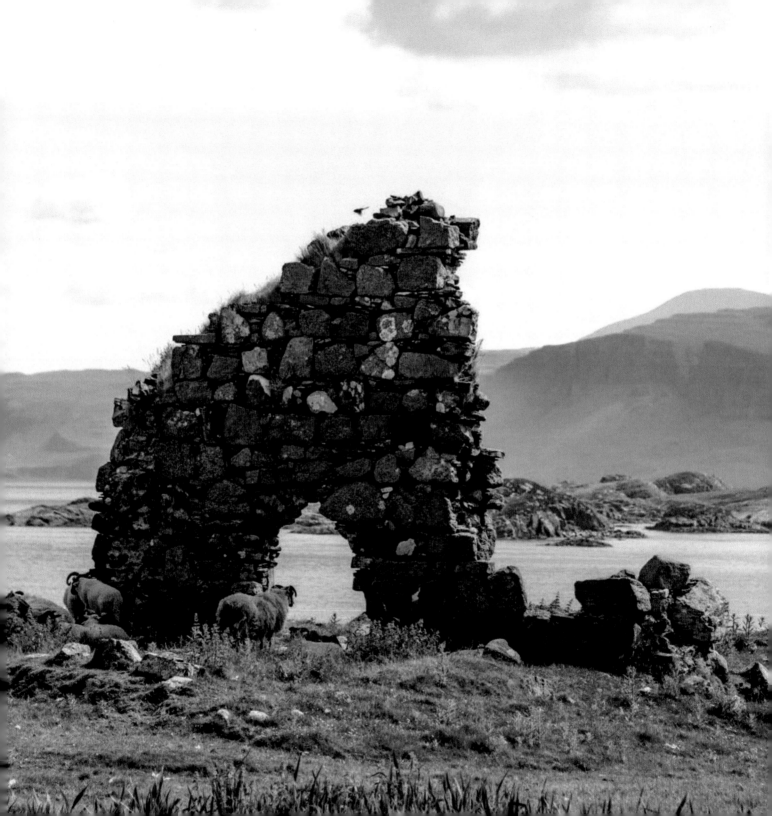

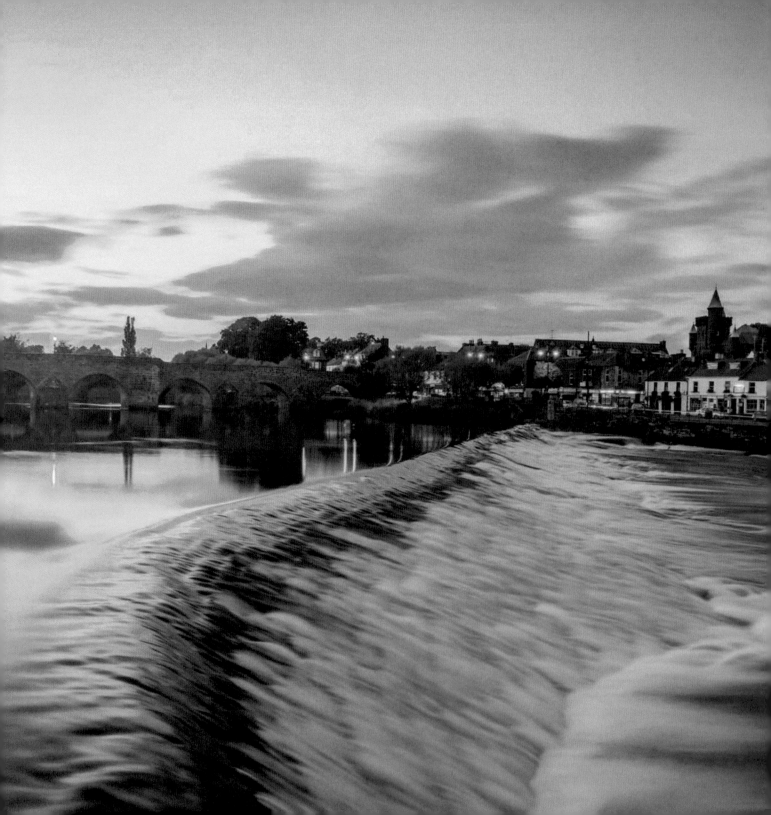

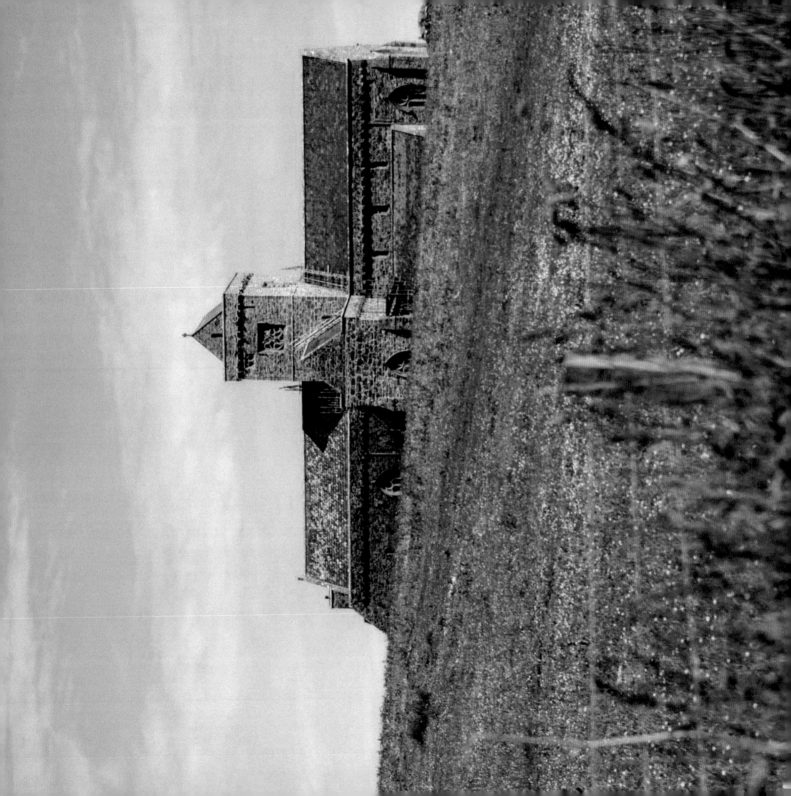

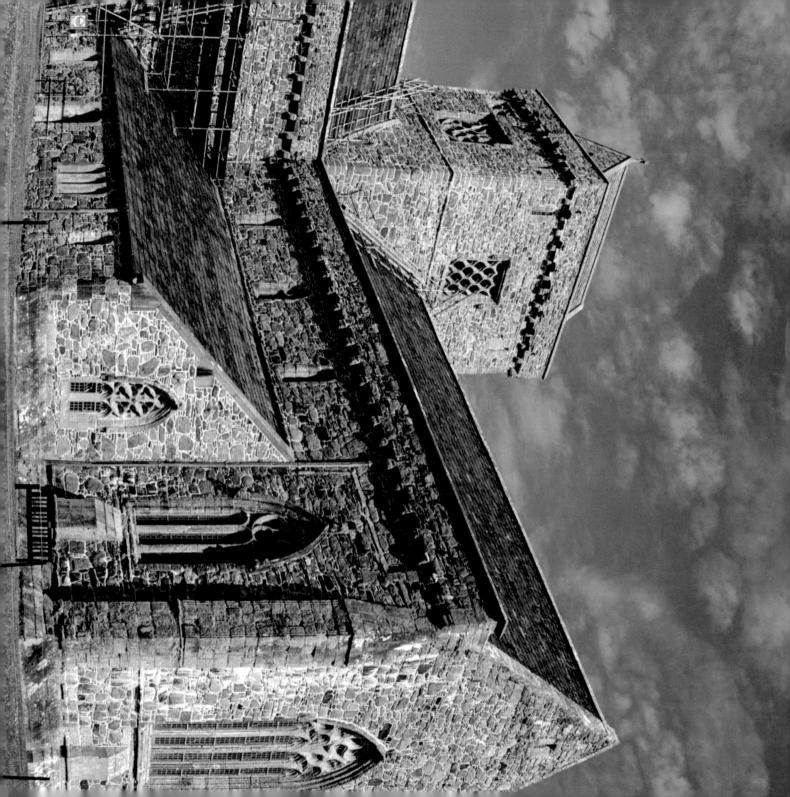